THE UN

THE KEY TO YOUR ULTIMATE POTENTIAL

JONATHAN BERMAN, MS
ERIN WHITNEY, MA

WITH DENNIS LOWERY

THE UNLOCKED SOUL
THE KEY TO YOUR ULTIMATE POTENTIAL

JONATHAN BERMAN, MS
ERIN WHITNEY, MA

WITH DENNIS LOWERY

ADVANCE READER COPY

PUBLISHED BY

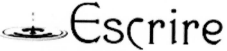
Escrire

A FICTION IMPRINT FROM ADDUCENT
Adducent, Inc.
www.Adducent.Co

Titles Distributed In
North America
United Kingdom
Western Europe
South America
Australia
China

The Unlocked Soul

The Key to Your Ultimate Potential

Jonathan Berman, MS
Erin Whitney, MA
With Dennis Lowery

ISBN: 9781937592547 (paperback)

Published by Adducent, Inc. under its Escrire fiction imprint
Jacksonville, Florida
www.Adducent.Co
Published in the United States of America

TABLE OF CONTENTS

Dedication & Acknowledgments

DEDICATION

This book is dedicated to the pursuit and Science of Universal Peace. It is also dedicated to my beautiful and loving wife, Erin. Without her help and support, this book would not have been written.

ACKNOWLEDGMENTS

I would like to thank my father Dr. Alan Berman for spending many hours discussing the physics of the ULE. His help was invaluable in developing the ideas addressed in this book. While this is a book of fiction, the mathematical theorem and the universal law it is based on are real. I would also like to thank my wife for her suggestions for the plot of the book. Without her help this book would not have been the book it is. Thanks also to my publisher for his expert guidance and work in producing this book. Thanks to the many people that read the manuscript for their helpful suggestions and criticisms. Their help was invaluable.

Since Man came into existence, we have been shackled.

In myth, Prometheus gave fire to Man and was punished. Though fire remained with Man, it could not burn through that which holds us back and makes us less than we can be.

There are a few that discovered how and escaped bondage and managed to slip the chains. You know their names—saints and sinners, intellectuals, geniuses, artists, and creators—but most of all who have lived and died... did so without becoming who and what they were capable of being.

Billions of people live today that will die the same way.

But they don't have to...

"That which can be stated without proof can be dismissed without proof."
— Sam Harris, in his book, *The End of Faith*

"Everyone is entitled to his own opinion, but not to his own facts."
— Patrick Moynihan

"That which can be stated with proof cannot be dismissed without proof."
— Jon Berman

PROLOGUE

The new boy felt out of place as blonde haired and blue-eyed boy in a predominantly Hispanic school. Most of his classmates didn't have the variety of experiences he had experienced growing up. There wasn't much common ground between them and as one of the smartest kids in the class he knew he wouldn't fit in anytime soon.

He had the misfortune of being in Mrs. Gonzalez's class. She was not very bright and would stand in front of the class and talk about her cousins and other things he found a complete waste of time. Initially, he asked Mrs. Gonzalez about subjects that interested him, but she seemed unable to discuss much beyond daily life. If what she said was ever interesting at all, it was only interesting once. After a while, he stopped asking questions and sat and daydreamed instead.

He would pretend he was sick so he could stay at home and read books. He figured that he would probably learn more that way than by sitting and listening to Mrs. Gonzalez. His mother knew he was faking most of the time, but she also knew why he

1

didn't want to go to school. It was during that time when he had one of the most significant experiences in his life. One of those days, pretending to be sick, at home lying in bed, he realized he would absolutely have to go to school the next day. The thought of listening to Mrs. Gonzalez was almost more than he could bear. He would rather be just about anyplace else than school the next day. As his mind perched on the border between sleep and awake he thought about school as a part of a greater reality, but what if that reality was one he did not have to stay in. What if he could change his reality and not go to school?

The room had become dim, turning to dark, with the sun now fully down and his room light off. But as his mind's thoughts carried along their path, the room began to fill with a bluish white light. He could feel it inside his body—something different—something powerful. It felt like an expanding energy and being part of it was both exhilarating and peaceful at the same time. The walls of the room disappeared, and he could just barely feel the bed where he was now sitting. He wondered if his mother would see him if she came into the room. Was there still one and was he still in it? Maybe he had somehow got into a different universe and another *him* was still in the real-world universe where he had to go back to school the next day.

His consciousness sat at the edge of different reality. If he let go of the concepts of time and space, he could leave the real world and not have to go back to school. But with that feeling he knew he would go on that journey alone and would no longer be able to see his father and mother. Frightened by that, he decided not to slip free from his day to day reality even though he knew it meant having to go back to school—the part of his life that he hated. As soon as he made that decision, everything returned to the way it had been. He was back in his room sitting on his bed. The thought of going back to school was still depressing, but that was the price he had to pay for being in this world. But he thought, if I did it once I could do this again... in a few years I'll be older and ready to take that step.'

Little did he know, his life unfolded and he'd forget about this moment. Two decades would pass before he recalled it and rediscovered the power to change his destiny.

CHAPTER ONE

"Man is the only animal that laughs and weeps; for he is the only animal that is struck with the difference between what things are, and what they ought to be."
—William Hazlitt

30 December 2015
Boulder Hospital

"Does anyone know how to turn this thing off?" The words, coming from the doctor who had just taken his mother off life support, were as cruel and harsh as the alarm's blare. The respiratory technician who hurried into the room shut it off and gave the doctor an exasperated look. With a button push, she had delivered what at first seemed like silence.

Michael heard the doctor murmur to a nurse who marked it on one of the papers on her clipboard, "Time of death 3:03 AM, 30 December 2015."

At different times before she slipped too far they talked about life and his future. He recalled Christmas morning. His mother's last lucid moment. She felt she was dying an unfinished person who could've been and done so much more, but life just had not worked out. Her last words to him were her final gift, *"Find the right way to live your life. Make the right decisions, now. Don't sell yourself short. You can be what you want to be... you can live the way you wish to live."* He saw in her eyes the unspoken words, don't let your life become like mine.'

She didn't deserve to die in pain; the end of a stress filled life and unhappy marriage. Opening his eyes, he watched as the nurses and the technician finished their work—they moved as a unit—the business-like clockwork of clearing the room. Unplugging this. Wrapping cords around that. Wheeling things into the hallway to get them out of the way. Whose way, he thought. But he knew the equipment, the machines, would be returned to storage or for use in someone else's life or death. The final, perfunctory, "Sorry for your loss," from the doctor; it all seemed thinly scripted and performed. No dignity. No comfort for the hard road just endured and no easing the path ahead. The soft sounds of their routine faded as they stepped out and the room became as still as his mother.

He remained at her side, holding her limp hand; he had watched her face and seen the last breath, a slight chest rise then settle... forever. In the corner of the room sat his father; head down. Glancing dry-eyed at him, Michael heard his sob, catching the sound in the hands that held his head. Face tightening, with thin lips he said, "You cry for her now, but she can't hear you. Your tears don't mean much. Being there for her, showing you loved her when she was alive, sure as hell would have meant something." Lowering his voice, he whispered to himself, "She was so much braver than you, dad. She never ducked reality."

Still holding her cooling hand, Michael recalled a vivid memory of his mother teaching him about bravery. He'd had a bike accident when he was eight resulting in a wicked cut on his right leg that required stitching. She had sat with him in the emergency room. When they saw the doctor and he had started to inject an anesthetic along the gash before stitching the wound to close it, she had seen he was close to crying in full. *"Michael* (always Michael... never Mike or Mikey*), sometimes things that happen in life are painful and we think they'll never heal, but they do. Even things that are torn or coming apart can be mended."*

He looked again at his father and that memory pressed him hard. Standing, he bent to kiss his mother the last time; noting how smooth her face now looked. The pain was gone. Feeling the grimace of it in his own face he wondered if it would ever leave him. The thought was interrupted. They'd come for her body. He released her hand, laying it at her side gently as if she was sleeping and he didn't want to wake her, and stepped away.

Jonathan Berman

Walking past his father's chair without a pause or a word, he stepped into the bathroom. Splashing cold water on his face he looked at his reflection. On his face, he saw his mother's eyes—usually soft brown, jumpy at times but often steady enough—now his own glinted hard as agate. He heard her voice, *"Find the right way to live your life."* His finely formed hand, with sinewy yet almost delicate fingers, used paper towels, pulled from a wall dispenser, to dry his face. He turned from the sink, walking out taller than when he walked in.

* * *

4 JANUARY 2016
OUTSIDE OF BOULDER, COLORADO

With the holidays, it had been impossible to get the service in before New Years. Michael had hoped to keep all the painful events confined to that past year, but his memories of 2016 would always start with her service and standing graveside on a bitterly cold morning of January 4th.

He was sitting on a bench, wanting to focus and burn as many details about his mother, the special moments with her, into his mind, but recollections of other things kept washing in. Like the tide; each had a rhythm and pulse that pounded its way to the front drawing the thought of her away as they receded and left him with a view of his eroded life. He shook his head. Four years of college, always scraping to pay his way, then years of meaningless jobs. Watching his family disintegrate as his mother died. What kind of life have I come from and where in the hell is it going to lead?

His chest was congested—a dead weight choke-hold on it from the belief that life was out of control and the unrelenting pressure would kill him. After the funeral, he had kept driving. No particular destination just hoping the automatic habits of driving would stop the spinning inside his head. A couple of hours outside of town, just off the interstate, he saw a sign—next rest area ninety miles—and pulled in. Sitting there he watched the people come and go—the transient flow—somewhere in between where they came from and where they were headed.

The same state trooper has come through before; this was his third pass, checking for problems or situations that might become one. This time the officer parked and came over, "Afternoon sir." The words came out in puffs of cold air. Michael glanced at his watch; he had been sitting there for nearly three hours.

"Sir, is there a problem with your car?" Looking at the **No Loitering** signs posted nearby, his real question was clear... What are you doing hanging around?

"No problem officer just needed a place to stop and think."

"Well, it's kind of cold to do your thinking outside... isn't it? Best you move along then to wherever you're going and do your thinking there."

Rising, stiffly from sitting so long, and heading to his car he knew the state trooper was right but didn't know where *there* was. He started his car with the trooper still watching him, he dropped it into drive, cranking the heater to its highest setting. When he pulled onto the highway, he still didn't know where he was actually going.

* * *

THAT EVENING
MICHAEL & LARRY'S APARTMENT
BOULDER, COLORADO

"Whatever happened to the guy who stood over me when Bobby Pinkerton sucker punched me?" Larry asked. "Made him back off and let me up." He looked at Michael, who slumped morosely on their couch.

Michael stirred, sitting up straighter, "What are you talking about?"

"I was wondering about you. I know it's tough. I still remember how I felt when my dad died and how hard it was for my mom." In the silence, he picked up the scuffed Frisbee they used as a dish to throw change into and rocked it back and forth, sloshing the pennies, nickels and dimes around.

After two or three minutes, it was more than Michael could take, "Stop it... you know that sound ticks me off."

"That's what I want. I want to get you really pissed off. But at yourself," Larry sat the Frisbee down, "not me."

"Getting mad doesn't do any good."

"Neither does feeling sorry for yourself."

Michael pried himself off the couch and headed to his room, "I've got to get ready for work. I can't miss any more days."

* * *

Work, Michael thought, dead end was more like it, as he punched the clock at the data center. One of the guys that had been there twenty years said once that this kind of job was what you did while life bored you to death. It was the same day in and day out. Year after year of 3% to 5% raises... but at least he had a job. Lots of people out there without one, he thought as he sat down in his cubicle and began his 9-hour grind.

"Welcome to the weekend...," he muttered to his reflection on the screen in front of him.

CHAPTER TWO

"There is no passion to be found in settling for a life that is less than the one you are capable of living."
—Nelson Mandela

8 JANUARY 2016
UNIVERSITY OF COLORADO BOULDER

Sharon Randolph's office was still bright and cheery with holiday decorations; the exact opposite of how he felt. But as his dissertation advisor he couldn't ignore her request. After the funeral and paying her respects, she had pulled him aside and made a particular point of meeting first thing Monday morning.

"Mike, I know how hard things have been for you and I'm sincerely sorry for your loss. But there's something that you need to remember. You're alive. And you still have life ahead of you. That's what I want to talk to you about, not your dissertation. Because frankly a dissertation and getting your Ph.D. doesn't mean squat when there are more important things for you to improve and focus on. Now, I'm not going to let you off the hook. I'll come back around to getting you on track with your dissertation, but we'll set that aside for later."

She sat back in her chair and looked at him expectantly.

With a sigh that was more of a grunt, "Professor, what do you want from me. What do you expect? I can't deal with anything, right now."

"You don't get it do you, Mike? Life's not about what other people want. It's about what you want and if you're willing to go after whatever that may be. Do you really just want to throw your hands in the air and give up?"

He shoved his chair back, "Why do you care... why should it matter to you?"

"I've known you and your father for years and watched what your life and events are turning you into. I also know what you could be... What your life could be. But you just won't let all the bad things and the negativity go. You're not trying to find a way to deal; it seems like everything that you're doing is just feeding them."

"I didn't choose my life. It sucks and that's just how it's turned out."

"Mike, sometimes shit happens and even the best people step in it. I'm trying to get you to think like a person who knows they can wash their feet and shoes. You can get clean. The crap you stepped in doesn't need to stick to you for the rest of your life."

He leaned forward, elbows on his knees, and cradled his head in his hands, "What can I do? I'm nearly thirty-two years old. I have a dead end job. My father is my only family and that relationship withered years ago. The one person I loved that believed in me is dead. Everything about me is dead!" He cried.

"You're not," Sharon stated so resolutely and with such heat that he looked up at her. "Your mother believed in you because she saw something you can't see for yourself. And I'm telling you right now if you don't give up and bail out on your own pity party... You will die and more than likely, you'll be miserable until you do."

She leaned toward him across her desk, "You have one of the brightest minds of any of my students past and present. If what you're doing, the way you've been thinking, is not making you happy... then you need to break the routine. You need to look deep inside and recognize that the only one that can make things better for you is you. Follow the logic and work out a solution."

Nodding, but not believing, he stood to leave. As he turned to go, he told her without looking back, "It's not that simple."

"Important things rarely are," she said as the door shut behind him.

She'd known Michael a very long time. He had started college with the idea he would be a physicist, just like his father. This was partly because he was very interested in how the world worked, but also because he wanted his father to be proud of him. The problem with studying physics is that not only do you have to be smart; you have to be willing and able to work hard. Michael had a lot of emotional problems that made it difficult for him to study. He had not needed to labor to get good grades at school, so he was unprepared for the amount of work in college. He failed most of his courses that first semester. The next semester was about the same. Eventually, he came around and began to get decent grades and to graduate with his Bachelor of Science degree and then his masters. Now he had a good shot at his doctorate, but he still had a lot to come to grips with before his life would straighten out.

* * *

His father was coming into the building for his morning class as Michael left and called to him. "We need to talk."

"You walked out on me at the hospital and barely said a word at the funeral. You've no right to act this way," he stated in a voice too loud for use while standing on a sidewalk with other people around.

"You're wrong Dad," Michael said, planting himself squarely in front of him. "You overlooked and underappreciated mom for years... she loved you. She asked you to make some changes. To make things easier for both of you but you wouldn't or couldn't—either way you didn't help her." Michael couldn't get any more words out and turned away. His father didn't have his usual condescending glare. Now it was naked, as if he kept him around to chew him out and feel above him because he knew inside he had reached his own limitations. But there was no audience anymore. Mom was dead.

Why did it always have to end up this way, each not willing to give in or acknowledge that it was okay to think and feel differently?

* * *

Robert Wharton watched his son walk away, stiff-backed as always. Shaking his head, he wondered for the thousandth time how life had turned out this way. It shouldn't have.

As he passed Sharon Randolph's open door on the way to his own office, he hesitated and then continued. The pause caught her attention. He regretted it the second he heard her.

"Bob, you got a minute?"

Sighing, he stepped into her office. "What's up, Sharon?"

"I just met with Mike. He's still not dealing well with things. How are you doing?" she asked with a concerned look on her face. She and Bob were both in their mid-50s and had known each other for more than twenty years—since he first came to Boulder to teach. She liked him, but they'd not grown terribly close over all those years. Something about Bob was standoffish but his wife, Sara, had been a lovely lady. She realized, not for the first time, she liked Sara much more than Bob. He seemed to exude an, *I'm better than most people,* attitude that rubbed her the wrong way after a while. Especially since she'd heard the phone calls through the wall of the office and knew his spending and financial decisions had almost bankrupted his family. She also knew he felt underpaid for his level of education and resented his peers that had gone into private industry where they made a great deal of money. He thought teaching was a much higher calling.

"I'm all right."

"I'm very sorry, Bob. Sara was a special lady. I'll miss seeing her."

"She was a good woman," was all he could say. Hoping to end the conversation, he turned toward the door.

She let him escape thinking that's the best he could say about his wife—he couldn't say something like, "I miss her, too."

* * *

THAT AFTERNOON
MICHAEL & LARRY'S APARTMENT

After tossing his mail and the rolled up newspaper on the coffee table, Michael sat on the couch. He faced the beginning of a long week without a clue on what he was going to do about his father and his life. He thought again about what Sharon Randolph had said that morning. The positive part was what she'd said about him being one of her brightest minds. But she'd given him a dose of medicine with the kind words.

He looked back on his life and sifted the chaff, which was pretty much its entirety. Picking up the newspaper as he thought he started turning its pages without actually thinking what was on them. It was a community newspaper and mostly ads. His eyes barely registered, glancing right to left over the words and pictures down to where his thumb rested on an ad for T*he Reader's Attic, Old, and Used Books.* Its logo was a two or three-storey house with a large square window high under a gabled roof. Framed in the window, backlit since the house was dark, was the head and shoulder's profile of a boy or short-haired girl reading a book. Under it was a quote and address. He looked closer and knew what had caught his eye: *Books let us into their souls and lay open to us the secrets of our own.'*

He remembered that quote from William Hazlitt. As a boy, at least once or twice a month his mother would take him to look for books. She called them their book safaris. They would get in her car and it was automatic; almost like the preflight announcement from the flight attendant, *"Put your seatbelt on,"* and then out came that quote from William Hazlitt. Every single time. He remembered asking her what it meant and she had told him. "Good books and good readers reveal two things. The one tells us of the writer's skill and within that skill is a piece of the author's soul. The choice of the book sheds light on the reader's soul and the hope they have in reading it."

Tearing out the ad, he entered the address into his phone, mapped it and got directions. It was in an old part of Niwot, just north of Boulder. He'd never visited that he could recall, though it seemed he and his mother must have visited every old bookstore in a 100-mile radius.

After getting into the car and putting his seatbelt on, turning the key in the ignition was like turning that memory over again. He could hear his mother saying, *"Books let us into their souls and lay open to us the secrets of our own."*

* * *

THE READER'S ATTIC
NIWOT, COLORADO

The Reader's Attic sat on a side street away from the trendy shops and stores – it did not look like it received a lot of traffic. He got out of his car and stood on the sidewalk. Looking at it he felt a familiar tingle and presence. Almost as if he was twelve years old and with his mother on one of their book-buying adventures. In the window up against the glass were three heaps of hardbacks with a small drift of dust and what looked like cat or dog hairballs around the base of the piles. The tallest, in the center, was about three feet high and with the window platform it sat on, the top book was at Michael's eye level. This center tower was crowned, above it in paint on the glass, with the word BOOKS in plain black letters with gold trim.

When opening the door, he heard a small bell above him. It's jingling was an old-fashioned announcement. Unlike the front window display, the aisles of bookshelves that started almost at the entrance were tidy with the occasional hodgepodge mound of books on a small table capping off each row. The sound of the bell hadn't roused a stir from deeper in the store. A serpentine trail of shelves and aisles led toward the back. While rounding one end table, his elbow brushed a stack of books, knocking them to the floor. He began picking them up when suddenly next to them were a pair of slender ankles in plain black shoes. As he rose with two books in his hand, he saw their owner was a small, slight woman with dark hair who asked, "May I help you?"

Startled at how she suddenly appeared he clumsily replied, "I'm just looking." He placed the two books on the stack on the table.

Looking up at him, tilting her head to the left as she did, she spoke flatly, "Most people are... The hard part is the finding."

Her tone seemed so devoid of the typical cheery *we-hope-you-buy-something* chitchat you get in stores from employees or clerks that he didn't know quite know how to take it. "Well, you've got quite a maze here," he shot back at her, "so the finding might be hard." Then seeing her empty right arm sleeve, he regretted his tone. That pang most people felt when they inadvertently did or said something insensitive to a disabled person. Starting to speak again, this time in a lighter tone, "But—

"Sometimes, what is the hardest to do, can become the best thing to do." She cocked her head to one side, almost looking sideways up at him. She barely reached his chin and the shoulder length hair that swung away from the lower side of her face was a blue-black sheen that seemed backlit even though there was little light where they stood. "I've not seen you here before... what brings you to my bookstore?"

"I saw your ad in the paper. It had a quote that my mother used to tell me all the time when we'd go out to buy books."

A flicker of a smile came and went on her face as she studied his. "Come with me," she gestured turning, "and let's talk about what you're looking for. Perhaps I have the book you are seeking." Following her it seemed the store got darker the further back they went but the blue glint of her hair never dimmed. He followed that until they stopped at a long counter, with what looked like the oldest cash register he'd ever seen sitting on it.

"Tell me what you're looking for," she said over her shoulder as she moved further down the counter to an opening, with a swinging half-door, and stepped behind the counter to face him.

"I'm not sure... I'm just... just looking I guess."

"Yes, you told me that but even those that are *just looking*—have an inkling of what it is they are looking for. Something I've learned is there is always cause and effect," she brushed her hair away from her face and looked into his eyes, "Our world is not so mysterious as to why things happen or why they are the way they are. There are things that move us and things that fail to move—physics and gravity are at play even with things as intangible as our thoughts. We just have to understand what the rules are, the logic of things and how they work and then we realize what to do to get the result we want."

She walked over to a shelf of books at arm's reach above the old desk that sat to the right of the counter against the wall. Without hesitation, she took down what was clearly an old, well-used but cared for, book. Putting it on the table and opening to one of the pages in the front, she read its single statement aloud. "When the soul sees itself as a Center surrounded by its circumference—when the Sun knows that it is a Sun, surrounded by its whirling planets—then is it ready for the Wisdom and Power of the Masters."

He wondered, what the hell does that mean, as she leafed through the book.

She continued talking, but apparently not reading from it. "Time has not altered most aspects of humanity or the human condition. Dating back for thousands of years we share much with all the people that came before us. Both our ancestors and those unrelated. We're born. We grow old. We die. And a desire for change to improve oneself is nothing new. That, too, is a constant human condition. But to change requires action. We have to be willing to face the effort and often frustration of making those changes... even when in the face of those who don't want you to change."

She cocked her head up at him again, "But perhaps you're one that feels different than the masses.

Maybe you feel there must be a better way. There must be a better life out there for you. But you can't quite name what it is and certainly are at loss on how to find it and make it yours."

Somehow, he thought, she's centered on something I hadn't been able to articulate for myself. I do feel different and always have. That didn't make me feel special. Mostly it made me feel alone; a feeling even stronger with mom's death.

"In this book," as she closed it and placed squarely in front of him, "is a whole philosophy of life. The total of the phenomena, manifestation, action, inertia: the qualities of force and matter in combination. These, in their grosser form, make the material world; in their finer, more subjective form, they make the psychical world, the world of sense-impressions and mind-images. And through this study, the soul gains experience and is prepared for liberation. In other words, the whole outer world exists for the purposes of the soul and finds in this its real reason for being."

Not really understanding what she had just said, he found he had opened the book without thinking. Looking down his eye caught another passage, he scanned the lines, and as unprompted as his choice of page had been he read it aloud. "The binding of the perceiving consciousness to a certain region is attention (Dharana). Emerson quotes Sir Isaac Newton as saying that he made his great discoveries by intending his mind on them. That is what is meant here. If you read the page of a book while thinking of something else at the end of the page, you will have no idea of what it is about. If you read it again, still thinking of something else, you will get the same result. You must wake up, so to speak, and make an effort of attention. Fix your thoughts on what you are reading— and on nothing else—and you will quickly take in its meaning. The act of will, the effort of attention. The intending of the mind on each word and line of the page, just as the eyes are focused on each word and line, is the power here contemplated. It is the power to focus the consciousness on a given spot and hold it there. Attention is the first and essential step in all knowledge."

He looked up, noticing he had leaned forward and bent lower over the book on the counter as he read. Her face was nearly level with his and showed the merest upturn of the corners of her mouth, "This book is for you... it's what you were looking for."

Not yet believing her, but intrigued, he asked. "How much is it; what's the price?"

"It's free but if you bring it back or don't learn from it that could be very costly to you." At his perplexed look, she added, "Sometimes value has to be determined once you've given something more thought—or given it a try. Think of it as a test drive."

"Who are you?" he asked and something in her voice made him add, "Where are you from?"

"I'm Indira and often it feels like I've always been here. Please take the book. I hope you enjoy it." She turned and went into what must be her office.

Michael stood there turning the book's pages for a couple of minutes thinking she might come back or another customer showing up might draw her out. Neither happened and with a sigh he tucked the book under his arm and left.

* * *

THAT EVENING
MICHAEL & LARRY'S APARTMENT

With his dinner from the Burger King drive-thru, Michael sat at the kitchen table and picked up his tablet to check email and some of the blogs he followed. Clicking on the email link with one of the latest posts led him to a website he liked and visited often. Today's post was:

"It's me who..."

Much of our life is eaten up dealing with external things that often create stress or worry. Like:

- the job
- the kids
- the car (that conks out after the warranty expires)
- the dishwasher (or any appliance that craps out, again, after the warranty expires)
- the bills
- the in-laws
- the out-laws
- not enough money
- not enough time
- not enough _____(*you fill in the blank*)
- getting ahead
- catching up
- *and so on...*

We do have to deal with these--and more. That's part of life. But often they begin to define us. They start to limit us. They become a reason why we aren't happy.

We all live in the real world (*though I wonder about some people*) and what I've listed above and more can be a real cause for worry. And that perception... the stress and worry... affects everything we do or don't do. It can make us feel like our life is spinning away from us... out of control.

But there is one thing that you can work on you have direct control of that will help if it is improved on. The following defines that one thing best...

> *It's me who is my enemy*
> *Me who beats me up*
> *Me who makes the monsters*
> *Me who strips my confidence*
> --Paula Cole

Working on *"Me"*; working toward incrementally improving your perceptions and belief about yourself and all the components of your life can make things better.

> *"There isn't a single one of us who has overcome the human condition of self-doubt. Whether you're a supremely confident person, a content Zen monk, a successful writer... it doesn't matter. You have doubts about yourself.*

The question is whether these doubts stop you from doing amazing things, from leading the life you want to lead."
--Leo Babauta

Setting his tablet aside, he opened the book Indira gave him.

CHAPTER THREE

"The solution to a problem is never found in the thinking that created it."

—Albert Einstein

7 FEBRUARY 2016
MICHAEL & LARRY'S APARTMENT

It had been more than a month since the funeral and Michael still struggled with the knowledge that his mother's life could have been saved if only things had been different for her if things had changed. Sara Wharton should not have died so young and not in the way she did. He was sure the toxic family environment created by his father that surrounded them for so many years—one she felt there was only one escape from— was what ultimately though indirectly, killed her.

She told me not to be mad... not to get so infuriated. And she's right. I don't know that I can solve my problems by getting angry... maybe I can't get mad enough to get it done. I just don't know, Michael thought.

She had hated and detested hypocrisy and hypocrites yet her husband, his father, had become

one—the worst kind because of his own insecurities—
and she had tolerated it. How could you live your life
with someone like that and totally subordinate your
feelings when it came to them? He shook his head at
how that must be so bitter to hold in. He'd like to see
all hypocrites hoisted on their own petard then there
would be less sour bile poisoning the world.

Michael held in his hand a printed page from
some website his mother visited. Across the top, she'd
written, *for Michael*. It was something she must have
planned to give him but hadn't. He found it with some
of her papers when he'd seen his father was not going
to clean out her desk, get rid of what needed to be
trashed and saving what was important. It had been
clipped to some other printouts she must have
intended to give him at some point. He unfolded it and
read:

WHEN...
You Stand

When shallow people, without original
thought and stoked by their ignorance,
judge or condemn you.

When fake people—focused on flash and
not substance—smirk at you or at what
they assume about you.

The Unlocked Soul

When the only one that believes in you, is you (or a few friends and family).

When you feel so different, scared and lonely inside.

And you still stand and face the unknowing or ignorant crowd and a sometimes blind and deaf world.

You give it your best shot... give it your all. Every day.

That's when the magic happens and your world (and perhaps that of those around you) will be transformed.

But it will last only for as long as you hold in your heart the strength and faith in yourself that made you stand up to begin with.

He put the page back in the folder with her other papers placing it on the small desk in his bedroom and then started dressing. It was another day to face.

* * *

THE COFFEE STOP

"What's that?" Larry gestured at the book in Michael's hand. He bent across the counter and cocked his head to one side to try to read the title from the spine.

"Something I picked up." Michael shifted it under his arm as he reached for his tall cup of coffee.

Larry was still squinting at it. "It looks old... What's it about?"

"I'm just getting into it. But it's about a key to life—fundamental logic about the single most important thing critical to changing anything in your life—something like that. I'm still trying to understand it."

Larry had topped off a customer's coffee refill before he replied. "Well, maybe you can use it to change your face... wait a minute. Scratch that... the only reason I let you be seen with me is because you make me look better to girls."

"Right. I see the girls just hanging off of both of us," Michael shook his head and started to turn away from the counter.

Sensing Michael wasn't up for a verbal sparring match, he gave him his patented Smart-Ass-Grin and left it at that. Larry had watched him draw even further into himself over the past couple of years with his mother's battle with cancer. Knowing him all of his life, he never thought Michael would hit bottom and just lay there. But that's where he was and had been for some time. He hoped that he'd see his friend spark to life again.

Taking his coffee and turning from Larry, Michael started to go to his usual table. Larry leaned across the counter and tugged at his sleeve before he got out of reach, "Well, we can dream can't we," he grinned again.

Michael headed to the table with the convenient power outlet by the big window. As he stepped around some people getting extra napkins, he noticed it was occupied. Miffed at that, he walked past the young lady sitting there to pull a chair out at the next table over. He didn't have his laptop today anyway. Putting the book next to his coffee, he pulled out a red pencil and a pack of orange sticky notes. He overheard, "No... no... Pearl Street is boring — seen that bought that... You know?" And the jingling of her bracelets as she reached for her drink — probably a double frappe crappy something. He was a plain black coffee type. She was pretty, though not as young as he had first thought; she had to be late-twenty-something but with a store-bought spa treatment look. Glancing over again, he noted the BMW keychain on her table. Not for the first time he thought, I'm thirty-one and what do I have—a clunker VW Beetle whose best days were a decade behind it.

His morning ritual thrown off by sitting at a different table, he took a drink from his cup, tasting the fresh roasted coffee, and smelling the freshly baked blueberry muffins—his favorite—Larry was bringing out of the kitchen on a large metal tray to stock the display at the front counter. He appreciated Larry's mom giving him free coffee and muffins every morning. She owned the coffee shop and had known him since he was twelve when he brought her son home from school with a busted lip, swelling nose and quickly blackening eye. It wasn't the first time Larry's mouth got him in trouble and over the years, in other incidents, it had dragged Michael along, too.

* * *

She had named it *The Coffee Stop* and twenty years ago, Mrs. Gilbert had been wise to pick this location. It was a bit of a rundown area at the time with the growth of new construction outside the city drawing most of the new or expanding businesses. That's why it had been within the means of a woman recently widowed. The insurance money and what she scraped together working two jobs for most of her forty years was just enough to buy the café. Its corner location on a busy street still had stable businesses to give her some breakfast and lunch customers.

She'd seen those companies go through some tough times and they took her along for the ride, but she got by and in the past few years renewed interest in the area and its gentrification brought her steady customers from the nearby upscale condos and apartments. The affluent young offspring of some of the wealthiest in the city did not mind spending $3 or $4 for coffee and the same for her home baked muffins. The recession had tightened the belts of most people, but the rich had money to spend. She didn't mind that they spent some of it with her.

She had seen Larry and Michael go through tough spells and each at different times had needed the strength of their friendship. Seeing Michael sitting with shoulders hunched leaning forward as if the weight of the world pressed down on him she came out from the kitchen to sit next to him.

"Mike, your mother was a fine woman and she's at peace, now," Mrs. Gilbert said as she sat down at his table. "I want you to know that you always have a family with Larry and me. If there's anything, I can do you let me know."

"Thanks. You and Larry have always been there for me."

"Well," she smiled, "a boy who stands up for my boy and gets knocked down for it... he's like my son, too." She patted his hand, never tired of remembering with pride her son had such a good friend. "Larry talks a lot like I need to tell you, and he's always after you to do this' or do that'... and over the years sometimes you listened and sometimes not. That's the right way to deal with advice, even when it's from someone who cares about you. But there's one voice you have to heed... the little voices inside your head and inside your heart... when they combine as one. You need to listen. It's telling you what you need to hear. What you need to do."

She picked up his hand and held it. He saw the tears pooling in the corner of her eyes. "Your mother always wished she'd listened to hers more than she did. I think she'd want you to learn from that."

CHAPTER FOUR

"There is no use whatever trying to help people who do not help themselves. You cannot push anyone up a ladder unless they are willing to climb themselves."
—Andrew Carnegie

7 FEBRUARY 2016
THE READER'S ATTIC
NIWOT, COLORADO

Indira had dealt with her own pain and grief. The loss of her arm hadn't been nearly as painful as when she was told her husband, son, and daughter died in the same accident that took her arm. That had spun her into an abyss of despair and the near loss of her soul. While climbing out, she learned what living was truly about. You have to face things. Denying does no good and hiding does not work. To live is to acknowledge the pain and the wrongness when it is encountered has to be either dealt with as best you can or if that remains unresolved, it will ruin what your life could still become. Many people live life blindly not knowing that there is a better way. Ignoring that light can be found because the dark is easier to live with.

"So it is written" she murmured to herself. Indira got up from the desk at the sound of the bell and footsteps coming toward her.

"I thought you might return," she said as Michael stopped at the counter. "How did you like the book?"

"I don't know. I've been reading it for almost a month now and some parts make sense and some of it doesn't. The part that's hard to grasp is when I try to figure out how it would work if applied practically and not theoretically."

"So you are a logical thinker and things must balance before they make sense?"

"Yes, in a way. And must add up..."

"And life must be relegated to numbers that align," she made a plus and equal sign in the air, "or equations that produce correct results?"

"Well, it's how I see things... it's how I sort things out."

"Are you an accountant who views life as a ledger... a balance sheet," this time she tapped the keys of the adding machine on the counter, "with assets and liabilities?"

"I just came in to talk to you about the book... not to get into how I see things," he said tartly.

"But the book is entirely about how you see things. You seem to want the book to be a formula. Something simple you can follow, but the good that comes from that book requires more work than that. If it cannot be distilled into that will you just give up?"

"No, but math is the only thing that works for me. It's something absolute and irrefutable."

"Are you a mathematician, then?"

"Not really, not yet, but I'm working on my dissertation in advanced math."

The pause, its quiet, was filled with hesitation—from both—she wondering why she should continue to try and make him see and understand and he about to turn away, frustrated again, leaving empty.

"So many have turned from the path. Just because they could not see the destination immediately." She felt too tired to get into pointing the way for him, but not able to help it.

"In the book I gave you—within its rational and logic—is a fuller expression, and it is so lucid that my comments can hardly add to it. But I'll try. Everything is perceiver, perceiving, or the thing perceived; or, as we might say, consciousness, force, or matter. The sage tells us that the one key will unlock the secrets of all three: of consciousness, energy and matter alike. The thought is that a person intuitively understanding their heart and the hearts of others is really a manifestation of the same power as the penetrating perception that divines the secrets of planetary motions or atomic structure."

Seeing the perplexed look on his face, she stepped forward so quickly he almost backed away though they were still separated by the counter.

"What you will find in the book is pure logic... it holds a universal law that cannot be disputed. Like gravity, the truth of it is always there."

She started to turn away, as if dismissing him, "Read further and focus on what you are reading. Then come back and we'll talk some more." She quickly walked to the door, to the left of the counter, into what must be an office, opened, entered and shut it behind her.

Shaking his head, he muttered, "This is starting to remind me of Yoda and that cave..." he left to go home and read some more.

* * *

A WEEK LATER
THE READER'S ATTIC

"This power," Indira said as she paced, "is distributed in ascending degrees."

He had returned better prepared. Sensing that, she had invited him to join her for a cup of tea at the café next to the bookstore.

"It is to be attained step by step. It is a question, not of a miracle, but of evolution, of growth." Pausing to drink some of her tea, she continued, "You love mathematics, right?"

Michael nodded and signaled with his teacup for her to go on.

"Newton had to master the multiplication table, then the four rules of arithmetic, then the rudiments of algebra, before he came to more advanced work. At each point, there was attention, concentration, insight; until these were attained, no progress to the next point was possible."

"Right. I know that. You have to build on education; it's your foundation to get to higher knowledge."

"Yes. But so it was also with Darwin. He had to learn the form and use of leaf and flower, of bone and muscle. The characteristics of genera and species; the distribution of plants and animals. Before he had in mind that nexus of knowledge on which the light of his great idea was at last able to shine. So it is with all knowledge. So it is with spiritual knowledge.

"Think of it this way. The first subject for the exercise of an individual's spiritual insight is their day—or perhaps more broadly, their life. With its circumstances, its hindrances, its opportunities, its duties. As an individual, we do what we can to solve it, to fulfill duties, to learn lessons. Most people do not focus and work at that consistently or with a plan. They do not believe or are too preoccupied with trivial things. To try to live each day with aspiration and faith is the first step. By doing this, we gather meaning and a deeper insight into life. And you can begin the next day with an absolute advantage, a particular spiritual advance, and attainment—you know a little bit more. So it is with all successive days. We pass from day to day, growing knowledge and power, with never more than one day to solve at a time, until our path clearly forms before us. It's always been there, but now it is no longer transparent."

As she sipped her tea, he interjected, "Okay I get that. But how do you establish the faith and belief to do that day in and day out? That's what's not clear to me."

She nodded, "That is one of the first hurdles to overcome. To overcome it you must have control. To learn control, you must overcome distraction. With control comes the perceiving consciousness that will lead you forward."

Seeing he still did not grasp the meaning, she continued. "Say some when an object enters your view and at first violently excites your mind it stirs up curiosity, fear, and wonder. Then the consciousness returns upon itself—reason settles in—and takes the perception firmly in hand, relaxing it, and viewing the matter calmly from above. This steadying effort of the will is control, and immediately upon it follows understanding, and insight. Here's another example. Suppose a man is walking in a jungle and a charging elephant suddenly appears. The man is excited, and perhaps scared or in terror. But he exercises an effort of will, perceives the situation in its true circumstances, and recognizes what must be done. Probably that he must get out of the way as quickly as possible."

She sat her empty cup on the table. "I know that is a simple illustration, but with knowledge the order of perception is the same. First, the excitation of the mind by the new object impressed on it. Then the control of the mind from within; upon which follows the perception of the nature of the object. Where the eyes of the spiritual person are open, this will be a genuine and penetrating knowledge and understanding. This is how our some of our most significant and life altering experiences come to us. In the beginning, with a shock of pain, realization or discovery. The soul steadies itself and controls the pain and then the spirit perceives the lesson of the event, and its bearing upon the progressive revelation of life."

He scratched an eyebrow and set his empty cup down. "So control of your life comes from the recognition of what the bad situation is, how it happened, and then taking decisive action?"

"That's it."

"Indira, is it really that simple?"

"Yes... but you know doing it can be difficult when there are always so many complex things going on to take our attention or that fool us into believing complicated solutions are the only thing that work."

"We make things harder for ourselves, don't we?"

She nodded, her blue-black hair, swaying, "And part of the problem is everyone seeks the quick fix—something for the here-and-now. Most people look for the easy button, you know like in the commercial on television. A shortcut to immediate gratification."

She stood and moved over to the window and looked up at the white bunches of clouds, with a sprinkling of them gone solo, exploring the bright blue sky. "You find you are on the right path when you realize it's important to live in the present, but we must live for tomorrow. The present lasts for only one second... one minute... one hour... one day. The future stretches before us to infinity."

"How can I find the right path, Indira? I'm tired of hurting."

She could hear the ache in his voice. After turning back to him, she walked to the table and placed her hand on his shoulder. "There are defining moments in life. A point where you can't take any more of the way things are. Then you must define a goal; an objective you must reach. It's that purpose that sets you on a journey you'll not turn from. That is when healing really begins."

She took a folded piece of paper from her pocket. It was a printed page from a writer's blog and handed it to him. He unfolded it.

"Half..."
By Dennis Lowery
(a little story for his daughters)

There was a young man, who grew up in a half-way house, lived on a half-way street and worked in a half-sized shop with walls painted hopeful colors.

He sat in the window of the shop each morning, watching the half-hearted people come and go and dreamed of a full life... one where there were two sides and a wholeness of things. Never cut short where he had to settle for less than all or what he dreamed was in the world beyond the boundaries of his small existence.

So he worked, he lived and wondered where his life would lead if he only followed that half-way street that seemed to lead nowhere... to see if it didn't.

What if he started walking--farther than he ever had before? Away from what his life was and where he existed--to where he could be all that he dreamed.

"Enough," he thought and stood up, walked to the door, stepped outside, turned right and was never seen again.

"It's a story he wrote for his children to illustrate a point."

Her voice made him look up from the page. "What do you think happened to the man... did he fail or succeed?"

Indira looked at him for what seemed a long time. "That depends on the man. He had to write the ending to his own story." She tilted her head still watching him steadily. "Didn't he?"

* * *

20 MARCH 2016
MICHAEL & LARRY'S APARTMENT

Spring had come and he had never studied anything as hard as he did that book. And as he read, it began to make sense to the mathematician inside. It was simple mechanics in a way, he thought, a universal law like gravity. It had the logic of a balanced equation, he summed it up as he pulled into the parking lot of the Yoga Workshop.

What he was about to do was something new. He had asked Indira if she would teach him some of the practical applications of what the book talked about. The breathing, stretching, and movements—the things that would begin to release some of the physical constriction that he had carried so long he didn't know how it would feel to be free of it. But the book promised that you could be. And more than anything, he wanted to feel free, again.

Indira hadn't wanted to take on that role, but she had known Richard Freeman and Mary Taylor, the owners of the *Yoga Workshop*, for a very long time. Mary was such a good, kind and generous teacher... she was perfect for him, Indira had said.

The entrance to the Yoga Workshop, from the street, was a dark red door, with a glass inset and the number 2020 in gold above it. To the right of the door a framed box enclosed information about the Yoga Workshop and class schedules. He stepped inside and immediately could sense this was the place to begin to work the body and mind together.

CHAPTER FIVE

"...the location of the body is much less important than the location of the mind, and the former has surprisingly little influence on the latter. The heart goes where the head takes it, and neither cares much about the whereabouts of the feet."

—John Tierney, NY Times

20 MARCH 2016
THE COFFEE STOP

The girl with the BMW keychain sat near the window, at the table he preferred, and turned the pages of a magazine. But she didn't seem interested in it and had a remote, troubled expression, as though her thoughts were far away. Michael settled in at the next table over, placing his book, a pad of paper and large coffee on the table and sat facing the window. The light slanting through the window profiled her perfectly; her face lit on the sun side and shaded on the opposite—the hair a sunshine blond and darker in the shadow. Her teeth flashed, beautiful, white and even, as she chewed on the corner of her lip. He followed the sharp line of her neck into the high collar of her blouse. Her contours matched the vista outside the window. Quite a view, he thought.

She noticed him studying her, recognizing him from her frequent mornings there for coffee and a quiet moment. Without another thought, she began to turn the pages not actually seeing them and thinking of other things.

"Wow, a couple of analogs," Michael heard over his shoulder and turned as Larry set a basket of fresh muffins on the table. The girl, hearing him as well, looked up questioningly. Napkins still in his hand Larry gestured at her magazine and then at Michael's book. "Analog." He grinned at both of them, giving each a handful of napkins and then returned to the counter. Making a pirouette, he called out to the line of people, "I know... I know... it's me you're here for and not the delicious muffins and coffee. Everybody will get their moment with me."

Michael smiled slightly at Larry's floor show, and glancing over, gave her a smile too. Watching her in the sunlight was a pleasure to acknowledge and not seeing anything in return, thought, she would be prettier if she smiled. Looking away from her, he gave his attention back to his book. But what should have been a passing thought got in the way of his reading.

When his mother died he had been at the point where he was so tight he felt he would literally die in three or four days—everything trapped inside was suffocating him. All the bottled up emotions he was afraid to deal with. They scared him. What if he prodded them, picked at them and rose up to explore and maybe find a way through them. Only to be overwhelmed and never be able to put the cork back in the bottle. He wanted so desperately to not be in his body; its skin and bone a canvas over cement prison walls. He wanted to claw through it but had nothing but fingernails and what if he did breakthrough—would what was on the other side be any better? So he huddled deep inside, seeing only the dark, and feeling only the cold. He'd been that way until he met Indira and began reading the book she gave him.

He sat the book back down on the table, stood and walked over to the window. The shadow he cast over her as he stood in the sunbeam made her look up.

"It's a beautiful day—just look at that sky. The clouds look like cotton balls right out of the box."

"You're blocking my sun."

"I'm sorry... just wanted to get some of it for me."

She made a slight shake of her head, "Take all you want," and with a final dismissive twist she stood with her car keys and magazine in hand and walked out.

* * *

25 MARCH 2016
THE BLAINE RESIDENCE
BOULDER, COLORADO

It was Good Friday and the clock on the mantel chimed 4:00 AM. Leather creaked as Natalie Blaine turned in the chair to look at the picture of her mother. It had been there for ten years; sitting on the credenza it looked over her father's shoulder when he was home and at the desk in his personal study. He still loved her, she knew. As successful as her father had been, especially as a young prosecuting attorney, he had always claimed the proudest thing he'd accomplished in life was her love.

Would she still love him today with the way he had changed? The power, more than money, had turned him into a different man. He was not the same man who, after her mom had died, held her each night and told her stories until she slept.

* * *

27 MARCH 2016
THE COFFEE STOP

This time, Michael was there first at the table in front of the large window. The morning sun slanted down so he tilted his tablet up to cut down the glare. It was a beautiful Easter Sunday. He heard a chair slide behind him and turned. It was her. She glanced at him as she sat, but again, just an impersonal glance. He saw the magazine she sat on the table. It had been doubled back to the article she was reading. He couldn't help but see its title:

Parents shocked to learn medical examiner kept son's brain-

"That's some headline," he observed as she took her jacket off and draped it over her chair. The comment didn't draw her out. But the Michael she sat next to was slightly different than the one from before. Nothing ventured, nothing gained, he thought. "I ordered some extra sun today—just be sure there was enough for both of us," he grinned and cocked a thumb at the window. That nudged her a bit; a hint of an upturn at the corner of her still silent lips. "You know," he continued as if she wanted him to, "I feel for the parents. I bet they were really pissed off when they found out."

She gave him a questioning look. "What?"

"That article. I'd be really ticked off if I discovered a medical examiner kept my kids brain."

She shook her head at him and saw a bit of eye roll this time. "But I'm not surprised." She looked up again, lifting an eyebrow. "I think something like that goes on a lot... on a larger and more dangerous scale. That's what worries me." But she still didn't bite.

"A type of brain theft I suspect that worries a lot of people. I consider the brain an instrument of thought used for rational decision making—among other things. If it's not used partly for that function—then it's no better than oatmeal in a bone bowl. If what you have is oatmeal, then it's as if someone took your brain."

It was as if she couldn't help herself, "I'm trying to read. What are you talking about?"

"It's your fault."

She gave him a cold look. "How?" she asked.

"That article. It made me think of something I've had on my mind since the last election. Something I think is very dangerous for people as individually and for the country as a whole."

"Okay, that sounds like it's more than inane bullshit and stray chitchat," she put the magazine down and shifted her chair to face him. "What do you mean?"

"What is going on is serious—severe even—and damaging for the United States... for want of a better term let's call it the hooligan element that's entered the political debate in America."

"Define, hooligan element," she asked.

"Those beating their drums—an unrelenting stream of hate and fear-mongering to play on people's fears (to get their vote or their money... or both—definitely both). After reading about that incident at a Rand Paul campaign event, where someone who disagreed got roughed up and a whole litany of other crazy things and statements from the far right, even now after the election. After seeing these things... I have to conclude that there is a significant portion of adults in the United States... that had their brains stolen without being aware of it."

"By who?"

"The hooligan politicians," he took a drink of his coffee, "and their followers."

"I take it you're a Liberal Democrat."

"No, more of a progressive independent."

She almost smiled at that, "How do you prove there is a hooligan element?"

"Why would rational people act this way otherwise? Why would adult men, especially trained police officers we expect to protect and serve us, attack, grapple, wrestle, whatever you want to call it... a person to the ground and choke them to death or shoot them without actual, valid, cause. By not legitimately without hesitation condemning these actions then the right-wing pundits including some within the Republican Party are saying they condone the behavior." He twisted a napkin in his hands and stopped when she looked pointed at it and then to his face.

"So you think that the Republicans are to blame?"

"No, but it's as if the Crazies have taken over – or at least they get more than their 15-minutes of attention from the media. I think it colors how we perceive people."

"What do you mean by that? You think that TV affects how people form opinions?"

"Of course it does but not at first. But if we're hammered with it enough—bam bam bam." Michael tapped the table three times with his knuckles. "Then it does affect your judgment of value."

"Sure, for cars and commodities... consumer items."

"Not just them. People... and places, too."

She looked thoughtful. "If a person or type of people is repeatedly shown in a certain way then we start thinking that they are precisely that without really knowing from personal experience."

"Exactly. We form an opinion based on what's repeatedly fed to us."

She leaned toward him, "If they—the media or a politician—label someone as being part of the thing — an organization or political party known to think the opposite of what they think — that believes other than they do; then are they really saying they don't matter?"

He hadn't been clear and he knew that was part of the problem; his and maybe society as a whole. "It sounded that way," He admitted. "What I mean is that in the rush to talk loudest we don't say what we should really say — we say things more dramatically — more colorfully. The better soundbite or tweet double quote." He shook his head. "We don't have a meaningful discussion to work through misperceptions. And that happens to issues too, like poverty and income inequality. Politicians say they have the answers but never really do. And because they play fast and loose with how the phrase things they can never be held accountable to reasonable expectations." He rapped the knuckles of his right hand hard on the table. "They, above all, should be held accountable to do the real work necessary to solve the problems we have in this country. Not just stoke fears and make false promises."

"Nice thought. That that could happen. But politics doesn't work that way." She brushed a strand of hair from her face. "At least elections — getting elected — doesn't."

"When someone running for office takes that approach, politicians from all parties should shut this type of support down. They should repeatedly and loudly denounce such actions—and more importantly mean it. And the media should step up and not give those that do something so unacceptable, all the bells and whistles attention—that seems to do nothing but turn into a feeding frenzy. News coverage should be about addressing the issues. Not providing a platform for errant, to put it lightly, behavior—scare tactics—and manipulation of people's responses by touching a live nerve. Something that's easy to do when someone doesn't have a brain to call their own."

She smirked, "Why don't you tell me what you think." Taking a drink of her coffee, she said more seriously, "I guess you feel pretty strongly about this. You think the people that pull their strings are the ones with the brains—and their own agenda. For them, it's not about what is right... it's about getting elected... it's about using people as a tool to get what they want."

He looked at her more keenly, seeing something more than the pretty face, "I'm tired of people being manipulated. I'm sick of feeling like things are out of control and nothing can be done about it." He took a breath, "I'm tired of assholes."

"Like politicians?"

"Them, too."

"My father's a senator."

He looked at her not knowing if she was joking.

"Really... he's Senator Carter Blaine."

"I'm sorry," Michael stammered.

"That he's a Republican politician?" she questioned as she picked up her magazine.

"That I implied your father's an asshole."

"Don't worry about it... he is," she rose to go. She was as tall as he and the sun glinted off her long blonde hair as she turned to pick up her purse and cell phone. Glancing at him as she walked by her heard her mutter, "But he didn't used to be."

He looked up and her lips quirked up at the corners in not quite a smile for him. Not quite. But maybe. He watched her all the way out the door and onto the street.

* * *

THAT EVENING
THE BLAINE RESIDENCE

She had loved—still loved the memory of—her mother but could never understand her; beautiful, rich and married to a handsome husband successful in his own career—she had everything. True her father had been fixated on his career to the point of neglect, but she had never heard her complain. There were always distractions and her lifestyle to occupy her time.

She had died when Natalie was ten, right when Carter Blaine's political career was taking off. It came on so quickly after the breast cancer diagnosis—it ran through her as is there was nothing—no one fighting back. It seemed her mother was empty inside or what had been there had simply gone, too soon.

The worst thing was Natalie felt she'd never told her enough that she loved her. And with that thought she wondered if she'd find anyone that she could love that would love her equally.

* * *

THE READER'S ATTIC

Indira pulled the chair out, "Is that a smile I see?" she asked, as she sat across from him, continuing, "Most people I know don't smile at tax time."

"I was just thinking about this girl I met."

"Is she pretty?"

"Yeah... but not so nice at first." He shared with her the conversation from that morning. "She comes from an entirely different world."

"Many people do," Indira sipped her tea, "but they still manage to get along."

Michael reached for the sweetener, "Well, I doubt we'll have much to say to each other if we meet, again. She doesn't strike me as my type."

"And what is your type?" cocking her head, she smiled at him. Seeing he did not seem inclined to answer, she continued, "Many people today are so busy inside their own minds that they don't let themselves live or take the time to learn to live. They may listen to their heart and mind, wishing for change, but they immediately ignore it or disbelieve that change is possible. They pass on what they hear or don't hear because sometimes they want something or someone to deliver their solution on a silver platter, through a filter predisposed to render an opinion without knowing the facts that matter behind what is being said or not said. For most topics, that's not a major problem. If you're discussing desserts, some like chocolate, some like vanilla... some like them both. You like the Denver Broncos; I don't like football, at all. Arguments work that way too. Emotional decisions... opinions... you get the point."

"So, what you're saying is that our minds can get just as locked up as our bodies, with stress and worry. All the crap that goes on in life."

"That's part of the problem. Important issues... personal communication need civil discourse—and we need to stop and hear each other out—as long as the conversation is based on facts—we need calm. What we have now is cacophony. Political correctness often goes too far. If people can't speak the truth of what they feel or offer their real opinion--then how do you have a meaningful conversation without it being a setup to manipulate a situation for a personal agenda?"

* * *

30 MARCH 2016
MICHAEL & LARRY'S APARTMENT

"Larry I've got to get away from Boulder for a while. It's been three months since mom died and my routine is so concrete—the people—the environment—I feel laced into life instead of feeling alive." He pulled out a sheet of paper with what looked like directions and addresses on it. "Mom left me a little bit of money and I put in for a leave of absence from work."

Larry put his feet up on the coffee table, something Michael didn't like, but after 946 times he'd given up trying to prevent. "Where you gonna go?"

"I was talking to Indira; the lady I've been studying with. She doesn't always answer questions directly so I told her I planned to take a break. Maybe get out of town and away from things." He tossed Larry a beer and plopped down on the couch. "Get this; five minutes after I said that she walked over to me and says, "A wet garment may be hung up and so dry rapidly. Or it may be rolled into a ball and dry slowly. Perhaps you must find a place where you are not rolled up into a ball. I know such a place."

* * *

30 MARCH 2016
THE COFFEE STOP

"He calls you, Miss Sunshine," Larry said as he set her order on the table.

"Excuse me?"

"I'm Larry," he grinned at her. "My friend... the guy who likes this table, too." Pausing at the blank look on her face but continuing to smile, "You know, taking all the sunlight."

"Oh. That guy. I haven't seen him lately. He seems a little intense."

"Well, he's had a rough year and things aren't so good for him right now."

"Is that why he comes across like he's one step away from snapping?"

"Yeah," he pulled a chair out and sat, "well he's working on fixing that. So should I call you Miss Sunshine, too?"

"I'm Natalie... you must work a lot because I see you every time I come in."

"My boss is pretty hard on me. I work almost every day and sometimes evenings, too." He shrugged, "It's a living."

"Ever thought of quitting and doing something else?"

"Nah. When you're your mother's favorite son... you have particular responsibility." Not seeing her questioning look, he kept going, "Of course when you're her only son; only kid for that matter, you get labeled favorite by default. But between me and you I'd beat out six other brothers or sisters if I had them."

She'd never seen someone talk so much while keeping a grin on their face. It was as if the words came out no matter how his mouth was situated.

"I don't get the connection. Mom? Work?"

"My mother owns this place. She opened it twenty years ago about a year after my father died. I grew up working here. I know coffee. I know muffins." He sat back with his arms crossed on his chest. The look on his face was like he'd just scored a point in some way.

She had to laugh, "And you're happy, right?"

"Yep. Pretty happy. I got my mom and I got The Coffee Stop."

"Is there a girl in your life, or are you a confirmed bachelor?"

"Let's just say the right one hasn't discovered me yet," he shrugged his shoulders and held his hands up making a can you imagine that gesture.

"You think they'll find you here?"

"They'll have to. Here I am and here I'll be."

"What about your friend, Mr. Intense? Is he like you?"

"Oh, no! Mike... his names Michael Wharton in case you're taking notes...," his tone became serious.

Jonathan Berman

"Mike is one of those guys that could do anything but can't get out of his own way. He thinks too much about the wrong things. About the why he can't instead of the why he can. But he's coming around. He's making changes and I can tell already it's all going to pay off for him."

She heard the admiration coming through his voice, "I guess you're rooting for him, then."

"Yeah... he's my best friend."

"He has an interesting way of presenting his opinions," she leaned back in her chair. "Tell me about him."

"I'll be glad to," Larry beamed.

* * *

THAT AFTERNOON
SENATOR BLAINE'S OFFICES
DENVER, COLORADO

"Was mom's death what changed you?"

"What?" Carter Blaine was at his desk and looked over his glasses at his daughter as she came in and sat down across from him.

"I remember your first campaign. You and she met with those women and minority groups. He seems so passionate about issues they faced — that whole gender and race equality thing."

65

He leaned back in his chair. "That still important. To my platform."

"To your platform..." Natalie shook her head. "I know it was important to mom back then."

Her tone made him straighten and take his glasses off. He set them on the pile of papers in front of him. "What's wrong Natalie?"

"I met a guy that I think I like."

She seemed uncomfortable, like a girl worried about telling her daddy she got a bad grade on her report card.

"What's that got to do with what you asked... About your mother?" He rubbed his eyes. "I don't—" the buzzer on his office intercom cut them off. "Yes, Janet?" He'd hope to get through his pile of reading without interruptions. "No, I can't talk to him right now. Tell him I'll give him a call this evening. Okay. Thanks Janet." He keyed the intercom, looked at Natalie raising his eyebrows and gesturing with an open hand toward her. "I haven't changed, Natalie."

She knew his mind was trying to shift back to the work in front of him. If anything her father was diligent in his duties. "The young man I met... It's just... It's just that he kind of reminds me of you before mom died." She rose putting her bag on her shoulder. At the door she stopped and faced him. "I'd like you to meet him and maybe you'll recognize what I mean." She shut the door behind her.

CHAPTER SIX

"The reasonable man adapts himself to the world. The unreasonable man persists in trying to adapt the world to himself. Therefore, all progress depends on the unreasonable man."
—George Bernard Shaw

31 MARCH 2016
LIBRE, COLORADO

The community Indira recommended to Michael was called Libre and it was ten miles up a dirt road in the mountains at 8,500 feet. It was a secluded, beautiful, place on the south facing slope of the mountains. You could look out to the south and see beautiful vistas of the mountains across the valley under the broad, expansive skies.

Spring had fully come and the view, Michael thought, being in the mountains and wide open spaces; looking out over vast horizons made him think about what Indira talked about: the vastness of the Universe. It gave him a more expansive perspective of time and space and the problems he was dealing with didn't seem so significant.

There was only one clock in the house, but there was seldom a need to know what time it was. Michael called it Hippie Mountain Standard Time. If something was supposed to happen at a particular time, it usually ended up happening an hour or two later. There were no television or computers there and a lot of time to sit and watch the clouds go by across the valley. After Michael had been there for a few days, he could feel himself relaxing into the slower pace of life.

Following what he was learning from Mary and Richard at The Yoga Workshop in Boulder, Michael spent a lot of time meditating, stretching, and just being. Sometimes sitting and meditating for two or three hours at a time. After a while, the space between each thought expanded and thoughts that did come up were calmer and less frenetic. It was a great relief to quiet the chatter in his mind.

After a week, Michael got to a point where there was only a tiny point of tension in his center. This center is the center of gravity in the body and is located about two inches below the navel. Michael had kept studying and knew in Chinese martial arts it was called the Dan Tien and in the yogic tradition it was called the Udiama Banda. That one point of tension was the only separation between Self and Not-Self.

The experience of having all but a tiny point of tension out of his body was an amazing one for Michael. He was able to do and feel things he had never been able to before. The most pleasant part of getting all of the unnecessary tension out of his body was his heart was completely open. There were no barriers between himself and other people. Because there was only that small point of tautness, there was no compression or distortion in his spine. The vertebrae were correctly aligned and floating on one another. His forehead was completely relaxed, and eyes wide open. Although he could move incredibility quickly both physically and mentally, his mind was silent and peaceful. He had never felt more alive and poured his newfound energy into writing down everything that he had learned from Indira, the book, and his own discovery.

* * *

14 APRIL 2016
MICHAEL'S FATHER'S HOME
BOULDER, COLORADO

Michael pulled into the driveway of his father's home. Looking across the street, he saw that Mr. Spearman still kept his flags out year round. For a moment he reflected his fierce patriotism. I wonder how many

Americans really felt independent and in control of their own lives? He shook his head. It was his first stop back into the real world he had to deal with facing the things he had spent so much time in Libre figuring out.

His father opened the door without any greeting. "Where have you been? I know we have our differences but when I hadn't heard from you in a couple of weeks and didn't get an answer on your cell phone, I went by and saw Larry. He said you were fine but would be gone for a while—you were working things out."

"Yeah, I needed to get away from here. From a lot of things, I couldn't figure out about myself and about us if I kept fighting with what's inside me. And if I kept fighting with you."

He looked at Michael and moved back into the family room to let him in. He sat in his mother's chair in the family room. From that spot she'd often smiled up at him and when things were heated and hurtful, words flying between him and his father, she'd look at him silently pleading to just accept his father's diatribes and not push back. It still felt like a battleground and took only a moment for the opening salvo.

"You could've done more with your life—you had talent—you squandered your potential. Look at you... what have you accomplished?" It was the same opening question leading to the same argument—the same start to the same conflict.

"Dad, I was the boy whose brain you wanted to flaunt and when I rebelled you felt I let you down. Maybe I shouldn't have fought you but I can't change that. I have changed who I am now. I became the me that was inside struggling to get out. We've been through this. What I came to tell you, now, what I want to show you is something different."

"What's different?"

"I am... what I'm doing is, and it's working. Don't take my word," Michael handed him a folder with The Universal Law of Efficiency written on the front in large capital letters. "Here's the math and my notes."

His father had that old look that don't waste my time hardening of the eyes, on his face. "What do you want me to do with this?"

Michael smiled at him. "Read the first page aloud to me."

"Seriously? Out loud?" He started to hand the folder back to him.

"Read it, dad." Michael held up his right hand palm out to block giving him the folder.

He harrumphed to clear his throat and held up in the light. "Some people have said that profound truths are very simple." He peered at Michael over the page. "This paper discusses a Universal Truth that has been proven by a mathematical theorem. The

Universal Law of Efficiency (ULE) states that all systems function most efficiently without unnecessary resistance. Since human beings are systems, human beings function most efficiently without unnecessary resistance. Most if not all systems, contain necessary, unnecessary, and inherent resistance." He stopped and lowered the page. "Do I need to keep going?"

Michael nodded crossing his arms.

"The Theorem..." he perked up a bit. Michael could see his eyes scanning ahead. "One of the values of mathematics is that it is a synthetic system that can prove universal truths given certain assumptions. The Efficiency Theorem (ET) assumes that there is such a thing as systems and that systems function more or less efficiently based on a frame of reference. Because mathematics is based on logic rather than empirical evidence, scientific studies are not needed to prove that a theorem is true. Once proven, a theorem will always be true, regardless of changes in society or worldviews. Because mathematical theorems prove universal truths, ideas based on theorems must be taken seriously. The ET proves the ULE, which applies to all systems." He was nodding his head. "Am I done?" he asked.

"Read the principles at the bottom of the page."
"Really?"
Michael nodded. "Please."

"The ULE Principles"

1. I will keep myself and other people safe at all times.
2. I know I have the courage to follow my highest values.
3. I choose cooperative rather than competitive actions.
4. I believe that all solutions start with the individual.
5. I accept full responsibility for my actions.
6. I am aware of and will release tension within my own body.
7. I will strive to reduce tension in all others.
8. I will reduce unnecessary resistance with my personal choices.
9. I will work to reduce unnecessary resistance worldwide to help others.
10. I will work to reduce resistance in all who I come in contact with for seven generations to come.

"Michael, come on. The part on theory was interesting. But what is all of this?" He waved the folder at him.

"You need to read it all. See what I've put in there and check my math and formulas. Look at them then decide for yourself."

* * *

14 APRIL 2016
THE COFFEE STOP

"He's baaacckk," Larry sang out, handing him his coffee. "Hot muffins coming out. I'll bring them to you and we'll catch up." He turned to go into the kitchen, calling over his should, "Your girlfriends been regular at your table—I think she came in just ahead of you."

Smiling, Michael turned and saw Larry was right. She was there, sitting in the sunlight. He stood for a moment transfixed feeling something, he wasn't quite sure what, but it seemed like hope.

This time she spoke to him first, "There he is, the Republican hater." She actually grinned at him.

"I wouldn't exactly say I hate them."

"Sounded like it," she pushed a chair out with the toe of her boot, an invitation to sit. "I haven't seen you around lately."

Ignoring the first part—why stir that up—he responded to the second as he sat, "I took some time. I needed to get away from some things... from here."

"Running from someone you pissed off with your strong opinions?"

"My mother died and I had, still have, some issues to work through. I couldn't do that here in Boulder."

"I'm sorry I didn't—" she stopped as Larry arrived with the muffins and sat down.

Larry grinned at her. "I don't believe you two have formally introduced yourselves so I'll do it for you. Mike, this is Natalie. Natalie this is Mike." Cupping his hand to the side of his mouth, in a stage whisper, "I got you fixed up with this one, Mike. While you were gone, I told her all about you," giving Mike a thumbs up sign and an exaggerated wink.

"That's all I need, you as a matchmaker... please shoot me now," and looking at Natalie he grinned, "No telling what this guy has said about me. Don't judge me on what he told you."

"Well, why don't you tell me, then, and I'll decide for myself."

She seemed serious and he dropped his smile. "What would you like to know?"

"Larry mentioned you were changing—for the better—tell me about who you're becoming." She paused to sip her coffee. "You can tell me later about who you were." She drank again and he thought he saw the curve of a smirk behind her cup.

"That sounds promising," Michael interrupted her. "I think." He gave Larry a look who returned it with an even bigger smile. "Well, that's gonna take a while... you sure you want to hear it."

"I know I don't want to hear it... I already have to live with this slob and I've got work to do." Larry got up with a wave bye-bye of the hand.

"I have a big cup of coffee and two muffins and all the sunlight so go for it," Natalie replied.

"Okay, then. While I was gone, I looked at everything I was unhappy with in my life: physically, mentally, career and personal. I took those, listed the priorities in order of importance, and created a plan for my life going forward," he looked at her to make sure she seemed interested in hearing more. She nodded to encourage him, so he continued, "The most important thing for me first was physical. I needed to get all of the unnecessary tension out of my body. I found that there needs to be some in your body to move and do things, but beyond that, tension is counterproductive. And I thought that getting all of it out of my body would have some significant benefits.

"I also realized that if I could get that pressure out of my body, I would be more open emotionally. For most of my life I had been entirely shut down—it was hard for me to express myself, especially to people I cared about. If I could just release what was locked up in my chest, I could be more loving both to myself and other people."

The look on her face stopped him. "Are you okay?" he asked realizing that maybe he was sharing too much. After all, he hardly knew her.

"Yes. But what you just described is something I've felt since my mother died," said Natalie.

He understood immediately. "It was my mom's death that triggered all this for me. I was tired of how my own life was so constricted. I was exhausted for no reason and so mad about how her life ended and how mine was becoming that I had to do something or explode."

"That's how I feel sometimes. I'm sorry I interrupted you. Please go on," she told him.

"Being in a relationship—any relationship—was difficult for me and I knew that if I could be more open and loving, then my relationships would be much easier. I remembered some of the women I'd met in my life. A couple of them I had only seen in passing and never actually met. I scarcely remembered what they looked like, but to this day I remember their energy. They literally glowed. I thought that if I could be more like that, I would be abler to attract a woman like them into my life." He paused to pick up his coffee but didn't bring it to his lips. He cradled it in his hands as if drawing warmth from it. "Since I knew how it felt to try to move and live with a lot of tightness in my body, I wanted to know what life would be like without it. I thought of the fluidity of great dancers and how they moved. They made it seem so effortless. I wanted to be like them. I also thought of great martial artists. They were able to do incredible things with their body, and to do that, you would have to have most or all of the unnecessary tension out of your body."

She had raised her left arm to rest on the table top and know that hand cradled her chin as she listened. "So what you wanted to find was basically stress relief?"

"Not just that." He shook his head. "It was far more than that."

She looked at him, cocking her right eyebrow, but didn't say anything. He worried that this would be where he would lose her. This was the part where Larry's eyes started to glaze over. He couldn't quite grasp it. The good thing was that trying to explain it to Larry had forced him to make it far more clear.

"I also, wondered how I could ever be as capable and intelligent as either of my parents. Both were very smart people—I don't like my father, but he's an ingenious and competent physicist... I can't knock his intelligence. I started thinking about how pointless rigidity in my body would affect my intellectual ability.

"If you look at pictures of Albert Einstein, you can see that his eyes are wide open and his forehead seems relaxed. Einstein said he thought he used about ten percent of his mind. Perhaps if I got all the crap out of my head, I could use more of my mind than that. A light at the end of the tunnel!

"It also seemed to me there would be significant health benefits. Needless strain in the body can create many biomechanical difficulties. If you have a lordosis, an abnormal inward curvature of the spine, which I did as a child, it takes more energy to walk and circulation is not as good throughout the pelvis and legs. That clearly was not good. So the logic was there. Anything that restrains you or limits expansion or full, natural, movement is not good for the body... and more importantly... it suffocates the soul."

Natalie was quiet but nodded her head. She knew that it wasn't just a body being restrained that smothered who you are. The mind and the steady beat of someone's opinion could do it as well. She looked at Michael's face and how his body moved with his words.

"Energy has to flow more freely in the body; I found it very frustrating and didn't think I could ever get it flowing as much as I wanted. I came up with an image that was very helpful during those first couple of weeks. I thought of a dam with a lot of water behind it. I thought of the water as energy and the dam as the tension that kept it from flowing. If there a tiny crack developed in the dam, the water would start flowing out of the fissure. As the water flowed more, it would increase the size of the crack, and eventually as it got stronger and stronger the water would break off bigger and bigger chunks and the dam would burst. All the held energy behind the tension had a lot of force behind it. The more pent up, the more power is needed to keep it from freely flowing. It takes a lot of effort to keep unnecessary tension in the body. That effort would be better used for other things. I wanted to create a crack and let what was inside of me take it from there."

Natalie sat forward to refill her coffee from the carafe on the table. "So what you did was to identify that you were locked up inside and then made a tiny hole to pour the energy through until the pressure released?"

"That's it." Seeing that she understood, he felt he had accomplished a major goal. "I had to visualize it so I could pinpoint what could be done to break through it. Another image I found very helpful was to think of everything inside me that I felt was wrong or confined as if it was a wall that I wanted to get past. If there was no way around it, there seemed to me to be only two ways of getting through it. The first was to continually bang my head against the wall, hoping to beat my way through, which would not get me very far and probably leave me with a bloody head. The other way was to take the wall down. This seemed a much better approach to the problem. I thought of the wall as the rigidity in my body or in my thinking that was keeping me from living the life I wanted.

"Most people are content to live within the walls that currently surround them. It doesn't matter if they built the wall or let others build it; a wall is a wall. It takes courage to move beyond our personal and societal limitations and boundaries. Those that try to go beyond them generally try to do it by bashing their heads against it with not particularly good results. I chose to remove the barriers, even if it was slowly, piece by piece so that I could have a better life. I viewed that wall as an analogy for all of the things that were holding me back and especially the avoidable stress in my body and in my life.

"I thought of my wise-assed friend, Larry and came up with a belief that reminds me of the necessity of moving beyond the things I've let limit me in the past—seeing them from different angles so I can see a way around or over them. You have to be a bit off the wall to get any perspective on what the wall is. A corollary to that is some people have more perspective than others. I've been told that I do!"

Natalie laughed. "That's an understatement." Her grin faded and she seemed more serious. "But it's like you said in one of our first conversations. We can't — you can't — let other people's way of thinking form our viewpoint. And it seems you found a way to take that out of the equation. The changes that I've seen in you elevate you above that."

Michael nodded. "It does. I'm working on how I can better explain that because I think it's very important that I share with others. We get so locked up inside that we don't realize buried deep within us is the key. That book I got from Indira helped me realize that it existed and all I had to do is figure out how to use it."

She looked at him and realized that as he had talked a glow came to his eyes and seemed to spread. He sat there, quietly now, but with the energy simmering just underneath the skin. She'd never met anyone like him.

* * *

THAT EVENING
THE YOGA WORKSHOP

Michael was working on his own after the class led by Mary Taylor finished. Squaring his mat in the practice area, he kneeled and placing his hands on the mat brought his body forward taking the weight on his hands and forearms. Perfectly balanced he inverted and brought his legs up over his head arching above him. In that position, head down and butt up, still supporting his weight with his hands; he lowered his legs with his left extended inside his left arm and the right outside the right arm and bent at an angle. Settling to the floor, left leg still extended, he gripped his right ankle and foot. Slowly he rocked it smoothly toward his head, his right arm now grasping the calf of the right leg as he gently placed the leg behind his head. Once there he easily twisted his torso, stretching further and settling easily into the position. Hearing footsteps behind him he unfolded to a kneeling position then squatted comfortably back on his heels.

"Wow!" he heard Mary's voice. "That's something you shouldn't be able to do yet—not even close to being able to do."

Michael turned to face her, "I've been doing some extra work... it seems so natural and easy."

"It shouldn't be," Mary shook her head. "I've never seen anyone do that so soon. I'd like you to talk to Richard and show him what you can do."

* * *

17 APRIL 2016
MICHAEL'S FATHER'S HOME

His father opened the door without saying anything. Michael came in and followed him to the kitchen. There on the table was a spread of notes on both plane and graph paper. Sitting next to was what he had left his father to take a look at. His father announced stood with his back to him and opened the refrigerator. "You want some juice or tea? Somewhere in here I think I have some of those vitamin waters." He looked over his shoulder at Michael shook his head. His father grabbed a bottle of water, shut the refrigerator door and sat at the table.

"What did you think of it?" Michael gestured at the folder in front of his father.

"I read it twice." He shook his head looking down at the folder and then up at Michael. "And I think it's pretty incredible. I haven't thought through all the implications." He shifted his chair closer and picked up the folder opening it. "And I've never thought about this before — with all the thinking I've done over the years trying to figure things out. To understand why things are the way they are." He shook his head again and held up the folder waving it. "This makes sense. All systems function most efficiently without unnecessary resistance. Okay, that's pretty basic. Fundamental, really. But what you've proven here takes it to an entirely different level." He put the folder down again. "Michael, that..." He pointed at it. "It's historic. Proof backed up by the mathematical theorem that what you call the ULE, is just that. As fundamental as the law of gravity. And we know that the fundamental rules of our world, such as that, they're not a matter of belief or faith — they are a matter of fact backed by science."

Michael was relaxed but also alert to something he'd not experienced before. His father's tone was of respect and even admiration. "Dad, I hope that you would understand. But one thing that's important to grasp and that's that the ULE might be even more immutable than the law of gravity."

"That opens up so many implications." He shook his head. "I'm not sure I follow what you mean and you didn't get into that in your paper."

Michael leaned forward and tapped the folder in front of his father. "I know I didn't. But all of that..." His finger touched the papers again. "Has continued to grow and evolve not only in detail but in practicality. I think the ramifications are so far-reaching that it may take some time to see exactly what can happen if an individual applies the ULE." Michael sat back his father's eyes hadn't left his nap too was something new. He was paying attention. "You know I'm pretty good at chess."

"You had the potential to be great." His father commented.

Michael smiled because he knew that to be true. "I think we, and by that I mean as human beings, not you and me, spend our life trying to live it with levels of tension that we are so accustomed to we don't even realize how they affect us. Since I started developing this." Michael nodded at the folder. "I can think more clearly and easily see six or seven, sometimes more, moves ahead in the game now. Think about this. What if we got one-half of 1% of the people in this world to that point? What would it do in terms of new ideas? Just think of what breakthroughs could be made in science and in arts and religion, as well. Everything the mind of Man touches can be improved."

"I don't know. You know people are. They're set in their ways, sometimes stubborn, sometimes lazy, and even like me..." For the first time since his mother's death, Michael saw genuine sadness on his father's face. "Like me... Thinking that they're smarter than everyone else that they can't figure out why things go wrong. Why they're so damn unhappy." Embarrassed, he studied Michael's face and instead of scorn or content he saw understanding and acceptance. He wondered at how changed his son had become.

Out of habit, Michael rocked back on the two rear legs of the chair. Something that used to get him yelled at by his father. He saw the look on his father's face. It flickered and vanished as he spoke. "The two things that help us make sense of our world and of our existence our religion and science. The ULE, at its heart, is the underlying principle of all the main religions. It's the goal of them to give people the system and frame of reference in life. In a way, that's the purpose of government as well. But the science of the ULE can be explained, and shown, to be exact of guidance that is the core benefit of religion."

"Michael, you and I have had our differences in the past and it hasn't been easy. You've always thought, that I've been too hard on you. And I have been. But it wasn't because I was trying to be mean or harsh. It's because I knew you had the potential. And I wanted you to grow up and be better than me. When I thought,

I was failing in making that happen... That twisted me in ways I didn't really understand until now." He took a deep breath and let it out slowly. With the ULE I think you've proven to me and I know to yourself what you're capable of. I believe that this is the discovery that changed your life. It has released that potential. This is something that you should also get into your dissertation and talk to Sharon about."

"I will Dad," He looked at his father who now sat with his head hanging down. He almost got up from the table to put his arm around his father something he hadn't done in a decade. He was about to stand and do it.

His father raised his head and Michael could see the tears in the corners of his eyes. "Michael, using that..." His eyes shifted to the ULE folder. He leaned back still looking him in the eye. And for the first time it was a look exchanged between equals. He squirmed in his chair as if trying to get comfortable. Or to prepare himself to say something he wasn't quite sure how to say. "Michael, can you help me change, too?"

* * *

18 April 2016
Sharon Randolph's Office

Sharon Randolph hadn't seen or heard from Michael in since just after his mother's funeral. "What is it you want to drop off for me to look at?" She asked him. "Is it work on your dissertation?" She heard background noise, a murmur of people and the clink of silverware or cups and plates.

"No, but it might become part of it. A new direction I think that has some importance," she heard him take a breath, "Can you take a look at it today and meet with me tomorrow morning to talk about it?"

"If it's something that's lit a fire under you... then absolutely. I have a meeting downtown today but drop what you have off at my office and I'll pick it up on my way home and read this evening. Come by tomorrow morning at 9:00 AM."

* * *

THE NEXT DAY
SHARON RANDOLPH'S OFFICE

Michael was there first waiting outside her office door when she walked into the building. He grinned at her as she shook her head at him while unlocking the door. Inside she turned on the lights, pressed the start button on the coffee maker her assistant always prepared before leaving, and walked into her office to the right and on the east side of the building. Hitting the switch for her own lights she set her purse and briefcase on her desk and moving behind it sat down and faced

Michael who had followed her in. Reaching into her briefcase she pulled out the folder Michael had left for her the day before. "Did someone turn your light bulb on?" she asked him as she flipped through his notes. "How long have you been working on this?"

"A couple of months." Michael was standing squarely in front of her desk.

She looked up at him. When he had called her— a big change from her chasing but never catching him over the past several months—he sounded different. Steadier, more sure, she thought.

He sat down in the chair in front of her desk, the same one he had uncomfortably squirmed in months ago and continued, "Something clicked while I was studying...." Seeing the look in her eye, "Reading on another subject not related to my dissertation," he added. "And what I was reading made sense, especially when I coupled it with math." He picked up the carved Aspen wood paperweight from the corner of her desk and rolled it from hand to hand. "I wrote it all out and that's what you're looking it," sitting the paperweight back down he gestured at the folder in her hand.

A beeping sound announced the coffee was ready and without asking he fluidly uncrossed his legs and in smooth motion rose and headed to the outer office. "Want some coffee?"

"Yes, please." He even looks different, looser, she thought.

The Unlocked Soul

Michael came back in with two steaming cups of coffee.

"Thanks." She took hers setting it on the Denver Broncos coaster on her desk. "Well," she repeated, "I'm impressed. This theory of yours," taking up the folder and reading the front of it, "This *ULE*, rings true on paper." Raising her cup and blowing on it to cool, she paused to sip some coffee and continued, "Your math is solid."

He walked over to the window and as he turned back to her, the morning sunlight fully caught his face and upper body. She had had him in this office more than a dozen times and realized this was the first time she'd not seen tautness on his face and neck, the tendons and skin stretched and standing out as if he strained to keep his head up. And his writing and presentation of the mathematics behind his theory surprised her with its clarity. This was not the same conflicted and confused young man from months ago.

He walked back and sat down with a smile on his face. "It's not just right on paper," his smile broadened, something she had never witnessed from him.

"What do you mean?"

"It works in the real world," he raised his arms over his head, spreading them wide, and she could hear the steadiness of his breathing and the strength in his voice, "it's working on me. I feel it."

She nodded. "I can see a difference in you."

Jonathan Berman

Michael leaned forward. "Do you have a few more minutes? I need to talk through some things about this." He pointed at the folder in her hand. "And it's going to involve my dissertation."

"Okay," she checked her watch and then her planner. "We're good for another 30 minutes or so."

He settled back in the chair. "In my Ph.D. dissertation, I want to use the ULE mathematical theorem to prove that all systems function most efficiently without unnecessary resistance. Because I have proven it with a mathematical system, there is no question that the ULE is true. And I've been thinking about some of the implications of the ULE. It's both a superset and the underlying principle of the Laws of Thermodynamics. You know that deals with molecular systems, but the ULE deals with all systems. This observation brings the study of all systems into the realm of science. People are systems, families are systems, governments are systems, and religions are systems. The world is a system. Because the ULE is the underlying principle of the Laws of Thermodynamics, and Thermodynamics deals with energy, it makes sense to think of non-molecular systems such as families and religions in terms of energy too." He paused to drink from his cup.

"I'm following you." She had a pad out and had jotted some notes as he talked.

"Once we can think of these systems in terms of energy, we can study them in a way that we've not been able to before. In fact, we can quantify energetic systems. And everything almost can be thought of as energy. If we can now quantify systems such as individuals, families and religions, we can study them in a way that we've not been able to before." He paused to set his empty cup on the corner of her desk.

She stood with her own cup in hand. "Want some more?"

He shook his head and continued as she filled her cup. "There currently exist universities that offer degrees in Peace Studies. With the discovery of the ULE, we can now legitimately talk about the Science of Peace. I am not sure how we would describe the energy interactions, but I would say that peace is the result of an equitable distribution of energy globally. Conflict is the gamble that an action will provide more energy to the aggressor in a conflict. Let's examine for a moment the concept that everything is energy. Land is a form of energy, food is a form of energy, money is a form of energy etc. The list is endless. People would presumably be less likely to gamble on conflict if they feel that they have enough energy. They would have too much to lose. People that do not have enough energy have very little to lose and thus are more likely to gamble on conflict. Once we understand the underlying principle of peace which is the ULE, we can start deriving statistical models that will more accurately predict whether there will be conflict or not. Since conflict is an exponential effect, predicting and intervening in a potential conflict situation sooner rather than later makes sense. It would take a lot less energy to prevent a war than to fight a war." He slowed as he watched her writing trying to catch up.

"It's okay—I'm getting the broad points—keep going," she prompted him.

"It may seem difficult to statistically model such a complicated model as Peace. There seem to be many factors that go into it. If we can reduce it to peace to energy distribution, that simplifies things considerably. It should be pointed out that there are now climate scientists. Certainly the atmosphere is a very complicated system. Climate can now be modeled because we understand the Laws of Thermodynamics. Since the ULE is the underlying principle of the Laws of Thermodynamics, we now have the underlying principle of Peace and should now be able to study it in a more scientific way. Conflict or global extremism or aggression of any type can be modeled by a sigmoidal curve. We see these curves in many of the biological and natural sciences. For example, the growth of a rabbit population will follow a sigmoidal curve. If you have two rabbits and they mate and have ten babies, eventually the population will grow quickly over a certain range. Eventually, though, that population will reach a limiting factor for reasons such as predators or lack of enough food to support the population. Because the ULE has been proven, we can now start to think about the science of universal peace. I use the term universal peace purposely. Normally when we talk about peace, we say global peace. Because the ULE is a universal law that is more immutable and more omnipresent than the law of gravity, we can now talk about universal peace. We can now start to talk about the Science of Peace. It may seem that peace is a nebulous and difficult goal to reach. That there is no real rhyme or reason to it. The ULE provides the underlying principle of universal peace. That is a large claim and needs some discussion. For something to be the underlying principle of universal peace, it must be both necessary and sufficient. The reducing unnecessary resistance is certainly necessary for universal peace. It would be impossible to have universal peace with unnecessary resistance. That would be like having an engine workings as efficiently as possible with the bearings too tight. That is not possible in ANY universe. It is also sufficient. If enough people understand the ULE and make all decisions based on whether an action will increase or reduce unnecessary resistance than universal peace will not only be possible but inevitable."

She put her pen down, stretched her hand and rubbed her fingers. "You realize this needs to put to paper and cleaned up—to make sure you can take the math and what you just talked about—so it can be explained where people will understand what the ULE is and the implications. Right?"

He smiled. "That's why I wanted you to hear me out. I follow it and I think you do, too. But maybe you can help me do just what you said. Clear it up so it can be concisely explained and understood."

Sharon leaned back in her chair, checking her watch, and looked thoughtful. "I've got a meeting to go to. But I think I can help with that. Let's talk this evening. Okay?"

* * *

EARLY EVENING
20 APRIL 2016
MICHAEL & LARRY'S APARTMENT

Natalie knocked on the door and when he opened it announced, "You have to go with me and listen to her," she tugged at his arm.

"Uh... how about a hello first?"

"Hello," she grinned at him. "Get your shoes on. You really need to hear her talk."

"Her, who?" he asked.

"Her name is Erin Watson and she's an Education Advocate. She's even worked at the federal level with the Department of Education and went to college with the current Secretary of Education."

"What's she doing here?" Michael smiled as he slipped his shoes on and bent to tie the laces.

"She's from Boulder originally and moved back here earlier this year. She's got two children: a son and daughter in the school system. She's pushing the school board to add classes in Logic & Rational Thinking to the high school curriculum. She's speaking tonight at 8:30 PM at the public library on Arapahoe Avenue. Let's go!"

* * *

PUBLIC LIBRARY

Twenty minutes later they pulled into the parking lot and saw quite a few cars already there. Easing Sara's BMW into a spot, Michael thought, driving this beats the hell out of my clunker.

Natalie shut her door and matched steps with him locking his arm with hers as they entered the library. In one of the side rooms, chairs had been set up and the front rows had already filled. They sat in the next to last row just as a woman stepped up to a podium and microphone.

"I'm Erin Watson and thank you for coming out this evening. I'd like to talk to you about something I feel is terribly important not only for our young people but more importantly for the effect it could have on our society, country and world as they get older. The topic, as you know, is teaching our children, logic, and rational thought. It's fitting that I want to start with an idea; something for you to consider:

"Everyone thinks that the principal thing to the tree is the fruit, but in point of fact the principal thing to it is the seed."

"That quote is from Friedrich Nietzsche. Now think about it for a moment. And I want you to hold onto the thoughts you had about the above quote. Now, let me tell you what I think (as you listen you may think this off the subject but bear with me ... it all comes back around to it):

"I think that in today's very busy world with almost push-button gratification for anything we need and the instant answer capability of the internet we forget that often the exact answers, to the critical questions we have, lay within us. It's what's inside that is important; not the low-hanging fruit that may seem to be the right answer. It's not the fruit it's the seed that's important.

"I believe that everything in the world, good or bad, starts with a kernel... a small seed if you will. A little bit of something that grows and expands until ultimately it becomes what it is destined to be or what it is allowed or cultivated to grow into.

"The kernel may grow from the elements and materials that it consists of in a predetermined way. And be driven by its own internal system or engine that takes in what it needs to keep it going. Like a tree.

"Some kernels are created as a by-product of an event and grow through its interaction or reaction with what is outside of itself. Like a stalactite that comes to being and grows through years of mineral build up from the ground water in the caves roof following the pull of gravity and dripping steadily year after year, to the bottom of the cave. Or an oyster's pearl that results from a reflexive self-protection mechanism; the oyster forms a coating around a grain of sand, to prevent it from irritating and abrading its tender flesh with a new layer being added year after year. And so the pearl grows.

"I think that human beings are grown from their own kernels. And what we become is both due to things we cannot control (but have to react and respond to) and those things with which we can exert some measure of control. Take control of those things you can and certainly govern your response and reaction to those things that happen beyond your control and make the experiences grow you the way you need and want them to. Here's some more food for thought." She motioned and the screen behind her was lowered. "Here's some quotes from people you may have heard of." The light on the stage dimmed and the first quote's slide appeared, pausing briefly and then scrolling to the next:

"You only have to do a very few things right in your life, so long as you don't do too many things wrong." - *Warren Buffett*

"There is no use whatever trying to help people who do not help themselves. You cannot push anyone up a ladder unless they are willing to climb themselves." - *Andrew Carnegie*

"We are defined more by what we don't know about ourselves, than by what we do know. Change offers us the chance to discover what we don't know and, therefore, helps us reach our potential." - *Mimi Welch*

"It's not so much that we're afraid of change or so in love with the old ways, but it's that place in-between that we fear... It's like being between trapezes. It's Linus when his blanket is in the dryer. There's nothing to hold on to." - *Marilyn Ferguson*

"He has half the deed done, who has made a new beginning." - *Horace, Epistles*

"The great end of life is not knowledge but action." - *Thomas Henry Huxley*

"Action creates changes, not talking about it." - *David Clarke*

The light brightened and the screen went off as she continued. "Climbing the ladder of life successfully isn't easy nor is it always intuitive. It requires deep thought on your part about your inner values, desires and determination to bring about change in your life. And a search and discovery of a meaningful outside influence or knowledge to help you get to where you want to be. It helps to study the successes of others to see how what they have done may fit into the framework of what you want to do. To walk the clearest, and cleanest, path to your goals as possible you want to give thought to what you want to do and find. And develop a plan that is the right one that will get you there. So take time for thought. Remember. You can't have the fruit without the seed."

She paused to scan the group of people. "I want us to teach our children how their thoughts, their ability to think and make logical, rational judgment are the seeds that can and will grow into the very things that make a difference in the quality of their lives. And that their life indirectly affects the lives of those around them. It's a ripple effect that can have far-reaching impact on our world today and tomorrow. Thank you for your time this evening."

As the crowd cleared out, Michael and Natalie remained. Seeing that the speaker was concluding her conversation with the last couple to leave other than them, holding Natalie's hand, he approached her.

"Ms. Watson, do you have a few minutes to talk further? I'd like to ask a couple of questions and find out more about what you propose for changes in our educational system and the impact on society."

Seeing the earnest look on the young couple, she replied, "Well, it's been a long day for me... but if you know a place open to get a good cup of coffee and a bite to eat I don't mind to chat with you."

Michael smiled warmly at her as Natalie hugged his arm, "It just so happens I know a great place for coffee and homemade muffins."

"Let me get my things together and I'll follow you. I've just moved back to Boulder and it's a bit different with development; a lot I'm not used to here. Just in case, give me the address and I'll plug it into my GPS. Nothing's worse than being lost in unfamiliar surroundings."

She had turned away so didn't catch what Michael murmured under his breath, but Natalie did. "No," he whispered to himself, "Its worse when you're lost and surrounded by everything familiar... but never again." Shaking it off, he smiled at Natalie as they stepped out into a bright and beautiful night.

* * *

MICHAEL & LARRY'S APARTMENT

"Do you mind if I come in?" Natalie asked as they pulled up to his apartment.

Michael looked at his watch. It was late and Natalie had never stuck around past 11 PM or so. "Sure. I just hope Larry's not laying around on the couch in his underwear. Trust me it's not a pretty sight." He smiled at her as he got his keys out to open the door.

The apartment was quiet and dark. Michael turned on the lights. "He must be out and about somewhere, but that's kind of unusual for Larry since he goes to work so early in the morning."

Natalie had walked toward the hallway then stopped and turned. "I told my father that you weren't like anyone that I've ever met before. But I lied."

Michael looked at her. She had turned on the too bright kitchen light and he saw her silhouette in shadow against the wall. He looked at her face and she was watching him as if expecting something but he didn't know if it was something that he needed to do or say. He stepped closer to her. "So you've met other men just like me?" He smiled at her.

"Many." She backed away from him toward the hallway.

He took two more steps to follow her. "How many and where are they?"

Two more steps and she was in the hallway. "There were so many that had so many good qualities. The things that all women want in a man and each one had one maybe two of those things. They're not around anymore... they didn't have what women really want."

"What is it they really want?" Michael stepped closer to her and she moved sideways down the hall.

"They..." She took another step down the hall. "Want..." She took another step and stopped in front of his bedroom door.

He was close in front of her as she backed against the door her hands behind her. He leaned forward hands at his side. She didn't flinch or move as he lightly kissed her lips, lingering with her taste. "What is it they want?" They were only inches apart. He heard her hands moving behind her back and the rattle of the doorknob.

"They want someone to love who is open and sincere. Someone who doesn't play any games with them and that they can tell when they're with them that it's just the two of them. Those are who we fall truly in love with." He felt her kick her heel back and open the door. As it swung open her arms came forward, hands on his chest and then around his back as she pulled him into the bedroom. "Michael, I've seen you change. I've seen how the energy flows in you. When you touch me some of it passes to me. I see how you look at me and that when you do that I'm all you see. Me. No one else. Not some other girl or thing. Just me. And I see how you care for other people and how you want to help them. You're all these things that have meaning to me and all in one man." She took him by the hand and led him to the bed. Turning she began to unbuttoned her blouse. "That's what I really want. You."

There was none of the nervousness Michael had experienced with his few previous nights with girls. Instead, there was calm and he felt something inside stir as he looked into her eyes and saw the same wonder and building excitement he felt coursing through his body. He had never held a woman in his arms that felt quite like Natalie. She was soft and firm in all the right places. She worked out regularly and it showed in the lift of breasts that seemed so full without being too large. Glad that his own workouts had started to put his body back in shape, he cupped her right breast in his hand and could feel the energy rise through his body— channeling into hers. Touching softly, with fingertips and tongue, he explored her body. He could feel her response—deepening breaths, a twitch, and shudder— ripples across her stomach and thighs that told him more than the moans of pleasure as his body and energy merged with hers.

After she had gone to sleep, Michael got up and started meditating. He didn't need much sleep. Natalie woke and went into the extra bedroom that Michael had turned into a study. It was dark, but she knew he preferred it that way. She stood in the doorway and felt something tear at her she had never felt before—she was comforted and happy just knowing he was there.

Though it was 2:00 AM and there were no lights on in the room, it began to lighten. She could now see Michael and the light were getting brighter. She stopped, holding her breath. She saw where it was coming from and it scared her. She entered the room slowly then kneeled by his side, "Michael?" Again, a bit nervously, touching his arm, "Michael, you're glowing!"

Opening his eyes, for the first time in over twenty years he thought of what happened that night when he was a boy, of the blue-white energy that filled him with a sense of wholeness, of being on the edge of where he desperately wanted to be and who he equally desperately wanted to become.

He felt it again and knew it would never leave.

* * *

22 APRIL 2016
MICHAEL & LARRY'S APARTMENT

The breeze was cool and fresh as Larry opened the windows. "Well now," he said seeing the smile on their faces. "Natalie this is the happiest I've seen Mike since Ms. Grant, our well-endowed 10th grade English teacher, didn't realize the top two buttons of her blouse were undone. And Mike had to go to her desk and ask questions—many questions."

"What a funny guy you are," Michael said, sliding a chair out for him to join them.

"We were talking last night," at seeing Larry's grin broaden, Natalie felt a blush threatening to bloom and continued. "Don't you think Michael should show others what he's developed? It seems to have actually worked. I've seen how it's changed him."

"I'm not sure I want to get into being some type of guru," Michael replied, "Not even labeled as one," he added not giving Larry a chance to answer her. "It's not who I am. I just want to get my own life straight. People have to be responsible for doing that for their own lives... I can't do it for them."

"That's the point," Natalie leaned across the kitchen table toward him. "A lot of people want the same thing. They want to be able to feel like what they do in life matters and they have some measure of control over it. Most believe that isn't possible or don't know how to do it. I believed my life was going to be what it had already become without much improvement. I didn't think there was a way to change until I watched what you've done for yourself."

"Being the house smartass, here is where I should make a joke, but I can't," said Larry. "Mike, I've known you since we were just kids. We've grown up together. I knew where my life was going and what I would do since I was twelve. My plan was simple. Take care of my mom and take care of this business. It's been different for you. I've seen you beat yourself up... rail against the man, your dad, and against what you thought were opportunities you'd never have. Regretting the life you had and hating how unhappy your mother was. You got to a point where you felt defeated before you even tried. That's bullshit. I knew you were better than that. Hell, I know you are better than that. And now you've figured out how to realize that for yourself. If that came through this book you read and what you've learned through math... then you need to share that with others, man."

"I don't know how to reach people, though," Michael raise his hand palm up. "Why would they listen to me?"

Natalie looked at Michael and he knew she would not let this go, "My father said something once," she placed her hand over his, "and I actually listened because it made sense. People will learn from someone who proves his message is worthwhile. People will follow you if you have conviction in your beliefs. Life makes way for a man who knows what he wants."

* * *

THAT EVENING
THE BLAINE RESIDENCE

Michael made a point of learning what he could before meeting anyone. Carter Blaine was an important man—a senator and right leaning conservative. Every move he made—every word he spoke—had an impact on those around him. He talked. People listened. On the drive to Natalie's he had a lot to think about. And how it factored into his feelings about meeting her father for the first time. The world is populated in the majority by those who adapt to the world. It shapes them and they feel they have little to do that can affect that. The movers of the world view things differently. The world does have an impact on them, but they shape the outcome of their efforts. They don't accept only what the world gives them; they reach out and grab what they want by adapting their world to mold it into their reality. His initial impression of Natalie's father was he was an extreme example of that type of person.

In person, he was even more impressive. Tall, about six inches more than Michael's 5' 10", an angular, face made up of sharp planes, framed by dark hair frosted at the temples. His lean but sturdy build impeccably dressed—not an item out of place or in disarray.

Michael, who never seemed to get clothes that fit quite right, knew what was coming. Blaine had all the marks of a hand crusher... and he was. Michael withdrew his hand from the grip and unconsciously realigned the ring on his right hand that had turned with the torque of Blaine's handshake. He looked at Natalie who was standing next to her father.

Glancing at her Senator Blaine said, "Natalie hasn't told me a lot about you—that's not uncommon, but you've lasted longer than others she's dated—that is unusual and interests me. I thought it a good time to meet you."

"You two chat while I get dressed for dinner," Natalie said with a smile for Michael and what seemed a warning look at her father.

"You have a lovely home," Michael did a three-quarters pivot to take in the large and ornate foyer, with an only slightly downsized version of a Gone-With-The-Wind staircase leading to the upper floors. Natalie was already at its first landing.

"This way and we'll have that chat," Blaine gestured to a set of French doors just off the foyer, to the left, as he faced the stairs.

Carter Blaine was the kind of man and politician who thought of his private office as a mousetrap. In his study, the gallery setting, artwork, and glass display cases built into the walls sitting on high are portrayers of conspicuous wealth that warn you of the owner's importance. It was all shiny bait to lure you mentally into the belief that he was a man of influence and means—a wielder or Power. And without doubt he was.

Blaine sat behind the over large desk with the scuffed leather top. It was roughed up the right amount to show it was a desk meant for work and not just for show. His hand, flashing with rings and wrist with its elegant watch motioned at the plush chair in front of his desk, not the one that sat at the side, which was a closer and more familiar seating arrangement. Probably reserved for those who passed inspection, Michael thought. Reaching into a humidor on his credenza he pivoted back while lighting a long cigar as his gaze rested on Michael. The smoke rose in wreaths around his head and collected in the corners of the high-ceilinged office like clouds on the paintings that populated the walls.

"Care for a drink?" he asked, indicating the wet bar by the windows that looked out over an immaculately landscaped expanse of yard.

"Bottled water, if you have it."

"Help yourself."

Walking over to the mini-fridge he felt he was being inspected, sized up. Over the bar was a plaque that read:

Jonathan Berman

PRINCIPLES

We, the Republican Party, believe in this platform and expect our elected leaders to uphold these truths through acknowledgment and action. We believe in:

1. Strict adherence to the original intent of the Declaration of Independence and U.S. Constitution.
2. The sanctity of human life, created in the image of God, which should be protected from fertilization to natural death.
3. Preserving American and States Sovereignty and Freedom.
4. Limiting government power to those items enumerated in the U.S. Constitution.
5. Personal Accountability and Responsibility.
6. Self-sufficient families, founded on the traditional marriage of a natural man and a natural woman.
7. Having an educated population, with parents having the freedom of choice for the education of their children.
8. Americans having the right to be safe in their homes, on their streets, and in their

communities, and the unalienable right to defend themselves.

9. A free enterprise society unencumbered by government interference or subsidies.

10. Honoring all of those that serve and protect our freedom.

11. The laws of nature and nature's God" as our Founding Fathers believed.

Scanning this as he opened the bottle Michael returned to his chair and sat, "Thanks."

"So tell me what makes you different?"

"I'm not sure I know what you mean, sir."

"Somehow you just don't seem the type to catch Natalie's eye... not that those smooth manicured young men lasted long with her." His eyes were dark and caught glints of light from the suspended light over his desk.

"I think she likes me for my mind."

At first Blaine couldn't tell if Michael was being serious or making a joke. "Your mind?"

"Well, I think I might be the first guy who could hold his own in an argument with her. Somehow that scored points with her and her with me." Some of Larry's smartass grin must have rubbed off on Michael as he met Blaine's look without flinching.

"What do you think of those Principles," he pointed at the commemoration over the bar. "You read them, right?"

"I did." Michael paused. "But, I thought there were only Ten Commandments."

"What?"

"The plaque had eleven."

"It's not the Ten Commandments, but equally important," Blaine's voice started to creep into senatorial with a patronizing undertone. "I believe in them as should all Americans that care about their country. Do you believe in them?"

"I believe in doing right by people."

"You say that like it differs from what I think or what the Principles espouse."

"I believe we need to teach adults to think for themselves and children how to think. So they don't get sold something they don't understand that isn't really in their best interests."

"What's on that list is in every Americans best interest," he tapped the ash off his cigar into a large brass ashtray, "the problem is the segment of the population that doesn't see things that way."

Michael sat straighter in his chair. "It sounds like you think the people whose beliefs don't align with yours or wrong."

"It's not about differing opinions. It's about knowing what's the right thing to do." Carter Blaine said.

"For the country?" Michael asked.

"Of course." Blaine rocked forward in his chair. "Michael, we have to acknowledge some people just don't understand what's needed."

"You mean they should leave the thinking to others. People and politicians like you?"

Blaine put his forearms on his desk. "I believe we are the proper route and means to make improvements in our country."

"Who decides what improvements?" He cut Blaine off. "And how will they be made?"

Blaine put his cigar in the ashtray and steepled his fingers. "Do you oppose change because it comes from someone other than who you approve?"

That made Michael blink. Resistance did work that way. "I think that decisions are made by a select few in power that have no sense of what life is like as an average middle to low-income American. They..." Michael swallowed. "I, like many people, struggle almost daily with problems and issues that need to be resolved."

"Okay." Blaine now had an interested look on his face. He glanced at his watch. "Let's hear them."

"And you'll listen and not tune me out?"

Blaine picked the cigar up and rolled between his thumb and forefinger. "Natalie likes you. When she told me about you, I wasn't impressed. But it was a change from her old menu of boys and young men she brings around. It didn't take too long for them to agree with anything I said." He gave Michael a steady look.

"Well," Michael met it. "I'm not like that. Will you listen... I mean really listen?"

He nodded. "I will. Might not — likely will not — agree with you. But I'll listen."

"Okay. First thing. Trust. Our political system is broken or at least in sad shape."

"What you mean?" Blaine had that look as if he was going to go into a patronizing explanation of how politics worked.

"It's polarized and sometimes paralyzed by big money and special interests," Michael said.

"There's always extremists in both parties." Blaine nodded. "I'll give you that. And it is an issue."

"But they shouldn't have the power to attract attention like they do," Michael said

Carter Blaine shook his head and this time it didn't seem as much at perceiving Michael as naïve as much as it was an acceptance that unfortunately that's just the way it was. And he did slip into defending the way things are as if they couldn't be changed. "Power and money, especially in politics, are almost inseparable, Michael." He shook his head. "I have to admit I don't like it when the one is so abused as to control the other. But it happens. We just have to do the best we can with the system we have to work with."

"I don't accept that." Michael said crossing his arms in front of him. "That very thinking is why people are apathetic about politics and we have such a low voter turnout. They just don't care because in their minds all the politicians think about is getting into office and staying there — not about doing the right thing for them."

Carter Blaine's face hardened. "You're young and don't know how the real world works."

Not biting on that, Michael sat silent, but already felt the tension build. Why in the hell did he let Natalie talk him into this meeting? She was twenty-eight, not eighteen and he didn't need to ask her father's permission to court her.

Natalie entered the room, dressed for dinner. "Are you ready to go? The dinner reservations are for 7:00 PM and we should leave now."

* * *

AT DINNER
FLAGSTAFF HOUSE

The waiter had just brought their coffee. Michael lifted his cup but not drinking, said to Blaine, "Senator, recently I spoke with someone, Erin Watson, perhaps you've heard of her since she's been to Washington to talk about improving our educational system." He took a sip and set the cup down making sure he placed it on the saucer that had accompanied it.

"I know who she is and I've heard her speak," Blaine commented, "I agree that there is much to improve with education, but I don't think the federal government should get involved. It's a state government issue." He set his cup down with a loud clink, "And I disagree with what she proposes as changes in curriculum... but again, the states should decide that." He sat back in his chair and looked coolly at Michael, who continued.

"Talking with her we got on another subject; how governments and political figures work the public—manipulating them to either *see* or *not see* what's really going on with their country or showing them how it was to their benefit to following party doctrine. Something she told me that I find interesting is that the average German citizen said they did not know about the camps. Right..." Michael gestured angrily with his fork, a piece of lettuce flying like a flag rallying the troops beneath it. "Erin told us that Nazi and German government and public records, uncovered over the past couple of years, are starting to prove that wrong. Many, if not most, of the citizens, knew and either went along like cattle or saw it as a way to gain something for themselves. They wanted someone to solve things for them... fix what had happened because of the Versailles Treaty and the slap down the German people took when they lost World War I. Well they got led... and along the way millions of innocents were killed."

"Yes, sometimes there are bad people—bad leaders—that do terrible things. That's my point. We must have strong faith in what made this country strong and can't let weak-kneed liberals ruin it."

"So you think that anyone that disagrees with you doesn't care about this country? That their thinking is wrong because they don't toe the party line?"

"It's not about agreeing. It's about what's right."

"What's right? You mean according to the people that bankroll getting politicians elected. The people that buy the outcome... their dollars dictating the thinking of the voting public."

"You're naïve, Michael."

"I don't think I am, Senator."

"Please," Natalie spoke quietly trying to get them to do the same. "Dad, you know how I feel. We've argued about that plenty since I turned eighteen. I believe a lot of people don't know how to think for themselves. And during election time they listen to who talks the loudest, no matter if it makes sense or not. The candidates that can scare people the most, about what will happen if they don't vote for them, are the ones that seem to get elected. That has to change."

"Natalie, we've talked about his before. How can you lead people if you're not strong? You can't. What you... and it sounds like Michael is a proponent of it too... want to do would be to give way to the weak."

"That's not it at all, Senator," Michael interjected. "What I believe is that if we had stronger individuals that would make for a stronger society and a stronger country as a whole. Individuals that are strong enough to be free of having others foist their opinions on them making them believe it's their own thinking. Individuals that are free from the limitations and constraints they've placed on themselves or those that others have saddled them with."

Natalie commented. "What my father is saying—and believes—is that you'll never change the crowd's mind, Mike, that's why you have to shape it for them early on."

He looked at her and then the senator. "I'm not talking about the collective public. I'm talking about each person as thinking individuals. They need to free themselves so they can think for themselves. I believe, I know, from personal experience, anyone can change for the better. They can leave behind old ways of thinking and of viewing life with a flawed perspective. What's wrong with that?"

Senator Blaine leaned forward. "My years of experience tell me people don't really change. Inside they remain the same. You'll see as you get older."

"I think if what's inside them is good and just and caring, then you're right." Michael wiped his lips with a napkin. "But what if that persona has been damaged? Maybe through mistakes they've made, but also because of events they had no control over. No matter how life might have twisted them into something or someone else, deep inside is that good person. They just need to believe the person still exists and can come to life again."

Carter Blaine put his fork on his plate with the loud clink. "Are you one of those types who sees the good in everyone?"

Michael thought Blaine's grin seemed sarcastic. "No Senator. Not at all. I do believe good exists but it's hard to bring that out and people that have had their emotional buttons pushed for years. By people who know how to use the media to do it to create a scared knee-jerk response that serves their agenda. It's almost Pavlovian."

"Now tell me, how is that the politicians fault?"

"You mean the people respond to that type of influence. Instead of tuning it out and making rational self-directed decisions?"

"Through the media is the only way to reach the people, Michael."

"It's not the how, Senator. It's the message and its shallowness. It's that unwillingness to believe you can even speak to them without the fear-mongering to control them."

Carter Blaine looked thoughtful and passed a hand over his brow, sweeping his hair back. "We need to get their attention. It's become the way to do that."

"That needs to change. We need to be comfortable enough with what we believe and propose that we can discuss calmly and respectfully and listen to all sides." Michael reached over to hold Natalie's hand. "Not everyone's the same. We all come from sets of different experiences and perception. But when a logical, irrefutable, solution is available — that's the right one — shouldn't we hear out all the details and then give it a try?"

* * *

THE NEXT MORNING
MICHAEL & LARRY'S APARTMENT

"What was it like meeting the senator?" Larry asked making his pronunciation of Senator sound like it came from a megaphone.

"It was like sitting down at an expensive restaurant to a fancy meal that looks great. Lots of colors, the right balance of quantity and perfect placement on the plate. Plenty of what food critics call plate appeal, but then you find out the food sucks."

Larry handed him a bottle of water and Michael took a swig, "Its Natalie's father so, after a couple of verbal volleys, I sat there trying to find a way to get my point across without turning it into an argument or debate."

Sensing a subject change was needed, Larry asked, "Did you meet up with John Wagner, the guy I mentioned to you who delivers our baking materials? He sure needs some help. I don't think he can keep doing his job with his back pain as bad as it is and disability won't support his family."

"Yeah. I'm going to work with him twice a week. I can't do it at the Yoga Workshop, but Indira has an almost empty second floor above her bookstore. I'm going to set up some space there."

* * *

THAT EVENING
THE READER'S ATTIC – 2ND FLOOR

On the wall was a chart that showed the relationship between applying the ULE and health. Like many pictures, it spoke more loudly than words.

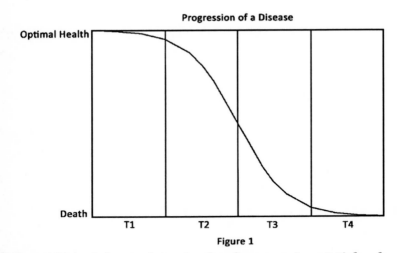

Progression of a Disease

Figure 1

It was their 8th session. At the first session, Michael told John, "Think of your body as a clutch that slips or doesn't engage correctly as it should. If it's not fixed something is going to lock up or burn out."

John understood that. It was mechanical, just like Michael said. When he started, he had barely been able to bend and even sitting hurt down deep, down low, in his back. He did not want to get cut on and he had not done very well trying to do the exercise his doctor recommended.

"Breathe in and visualize your body as a container holding everything in—the air in your lungs... your muscles... your thoughts... everything." Michael's whole stance tensed and his entire body went rigid. "Then let it go." He could see Michael relax.

"One thing at a time. Exhale slowly. Focus on each muscle and tell it to relax. You're in control. Let your thoughts float. Don't fixate on the pain. The worry. Believe in your heart and soul that freedom is there for everyone. We just need to let ourselves attain it."

John pictured his body as a machine whose parts had stiffened and rusted, then saw in his mind his hand lubricating the wheels, dislodging bits of dirt and metal that were blocking their turn and rotation. As each obstruction and impediment was removed in his mind, he felt his body loosen and felt that energy running through his muscles. He bent at the waist, not flexing his knees, and touched his palms flat on the floor. Not a bit of pain. He looked up at Michael a grin spanning his face; it matched the one on Michael's.

The next week John brought his wife. The week after, two friends joined the group. Soon over a hundred people had approached Michael to help them and it grew every day. It was all a result of word of mouth.

* * *

29 APRIL 2016
MICHAEL & LARRY'S APARTMENT

"You could do an infomercial," Larry said excitedly. "I know a guy who says he knows a guy in advertising that worked for Tony Robbins... you know... the walk on fire guy that's on TV."

"You know a guy who knows a guy who says he knows a guy... Right, Larry." Michael laughed. "I'm not doing an infomercial," he said seriously coming back from the kitchen with their drinks. "That's not who I want to be or how I want to come across to people."

"How you gonna reach more people then... wait! You could start a church. There's..."

"No way!" Michael stopped him. "I'm not going to preach this and make it out to be religion. It's not."

"But there's tax advant--"

"No, Larry!"

"I could be a deacon or something with cool robes that--"

"NO! Stop with the crazy ideas, Larry."

"Well, what about a school or seminars?"

"That could work," Michael agreed. "It would be slow, but it's a start. I wish there were a faster way to get the word out, though."

"There is." Natalie had been quiet. Michael and Larry looked at her. "There is a faster and better way," she said more pointedly. "What's the thing that draws a lot of media attention and public discussion—more than religion—more than sex?"

"Sports!"

"Larry!" both Natalie and Michael cried, then all three laughed.

"Politics," Natalie continued. "It used to come in its own season—the election cycle—now it's year round. And the last few years the public has had a steady diet of it."

"Yeah... I'm full of it because the politicians are full of it," said Larry.

Michael sat silently, looking at Natalie, having an idea of where she was headed with the discussion and already not liking it.

She returned his look, "What if someone ran for office—for senator—that was an actual anti-politician?"

"What does that mean?" Michael asked eyeing her intently.

"It means a candidate not tied to a political party belief system—no party line or special interest agenda. Someone who thinks politics, as we know it, is broken. And the only players in the game, right now, the backers of that flawed system, are those who gain from it. A candidate, who knows, at a deeply personal level, how to overcome internal obstacles, especially those that seem endemic. Someone who is not afraid to be different when that's what is needed for the common good."

Larry's grin was dialed up to eleven as Natalie smiled sweetly at Michael, "Someone who believes politicians today, are assholes and the public deserves better."

"Me?" Michael squirmed in his seat, "That's ridiculous, Natalie, I don't have any money and don't know how to go about raising it. There's not enough time. Your father even mentioned the elections not that far off—he sounded like he was sure he had it sewn up."

She had that clench to her jaw that he had learned meant she was going to dig in to make her point. "He believes he'll win because no one is running against him... unless..."

"You're talking about a lot of money and people to run a campaign. I don't know anyone who has that kind of cash or knows how to even get started."

"Oh, yes you do... me."

* * *

THE NEXT MORNING
THE BLAINE RESIDENCE

"Your boyfriend is going to do what?" scoffed Carter Blaine. "Who gave him that idea?"

"I did," said Natalie, not flinching.

"He's crazy or stupid to take you up on that," he snapped, "He's a done nothing nobody. No one will back him... there's no way he has the money..."

"I will and I do. I have my trust fund."

"Natalie, have you lost your mind? What is wrong with you?

"I'd rather spend it on something worthwhile. Something that can help others instead of on shopping trips to Europe or skiing vacations to Davos."

"You'll burn through your $10 million for a losing cause and end up with nothing. Then what?" He didn't wait for her reply, "Natalie, don't do this to yourself. He can't beat me."

"Even if he doesn't it will prove a point... one that needs to be made."

"What point?"

"That things can change for the better. That people can change."

"You have everything anyone could possibly want. What is there to change?"

"You don't know me."

"Why are you doing this... why with this young man that you hardly know?"

"Michael makes me feel good. Like I can make a difference... a positive one. Others need to feel the same way and he can help them do it."

"I don't understand," he shook his head.

"I know—that's why I need to do this." She had been leaning on his credenza with him turned toward her as they talked. She knelt by his chair and took his hand. "Who knows, dad. Maybe you can learn something from Michael."

* * *

EVENING
30 APRIL 2016
THE READER'S ATTIC —2ND FLOOR

They had met to talk about what Michael was considering: running for the Senate against Natalie's father.

"He can outspend you," Natalie said. "I don't have the kind of money his backers, the Forche brothers, are willing to spend—they see my dad as the next GOP president." She paused; Michael had told her how reluctant he had been all his life to ask anyone for help. He wouldn't be comfortable with what she was going to propose.

"You have friends, and friends of friends who feel something needs to be done to make their life—the next thirty, forty, fifty or sixty years they'll live and raise families in—better and more balanced with equitable opportunities. That makes up a world of people who want change. They want to believe in and help someone who plans to do the right things for them and this country."

"Yeah, I'm sure they're just going to rush to help," Michael commented Half-serious, half-joking.

"They will," Natalie insisted, "if you talk to them like you know you can. Let them feel the energy in you—like you shared with me, Larry, your father, and others we know. They'll believe in your message."

"Right. They'll join the club. A fan club for Michael Wharton."

"No, not a bunch of fans of you, just the beginning of what hopefully will be an organization of people who change the world one person at a time."

"You think they'll believe me."

"Yes, they will. I did."

She stood and walked over to him. "I've been around every one of my father's campaigns since I was nine years old. My degree is in Political Science though I've never used it. I know people that can help do this."

"But I don't know if I can do this," Michael replied.

"He's not going to take you seriously—and by the time he realizes he should it'll be too late to beat us," Natalie reached over to put her hand on his arm.

"In the best of times and the worst of times we are kept company with two things: how we perceive our self and how others perceive us. Too many people worry about the latter and not the former." Indira turned from the window to face Michael and Natalie, "We see so much of the bright shiny people that occupy the media spotlight and attention. Many with little of substance or real worth behind their perfect smiles. One wonders what they see when they look at their reflection. Even those that seem graced with fortune are often haunted in some way."

Seeing Michael still uncertain, she continued, "I saw you change yourself, Michael and I see how that has affected your friends in a good way. I see Natalie reaching from within to be more than she was before. To do more than she has in the past. That is something you do not do unless what you've kept inside is important enough to act on."

Michael stood and began pacing, "Probably the most important thing I've learned from you, Indira, is that it's how you feel about yourself that dictates the shape of your life. You can choose to live life honestly, unrestrained, and not give into perception or conform to the opinions of others without thinking for yourself—without doing what you need to do to solve your own problems and remove the limitations you set for yourself."

"That's true," said Indira. "So much of life is dictated by the quality of what we think and that will only improve with the stopping of false thoughts and elimination of belief in things that can be proven wrong or that are inaccurate. We must base our thinking on truth and facts; colored only by emotions driven by inclusive and positive beliefs—not bigoted and negative ones. We are creatures of habit and routine and often need something to prompt us to consider our thoughts... to provoke their evaluation and what forms or has formed them. And to weigh it all in balance so choices can be made."

Looking at Natalie, Michael said, "When I met your father the first time, I told him that you liked me for my mind," he smiled. "I didn't tell him that I had to learn to shape my life so I could look in the mirror and smile proudly at who was looking back at me before you'd have given me the time of day. Let's do this. Let's see if I can reach the people."

* * *

1 JUNE 2016
MICHAEL'S CAMPAIGN OFFICE

Getting on the ticket was the kind of paperwork avalanche and getting an office setup and staff lined up was work on a scale he had never imagined. Without Natalie's experience with her father's campaign's and her resources, it would have been impossible to deal with and get done. Larry's idea for ads that didn't look like any political ads ever created worked. They began to draw people to hear him speak. It was just small crowds at first; a dozen or so at *The Coffee Stop* and other places. Then more... hundreds of people each time. Michael learned to speak to the people's desire for simple communication. He talked about issues and not agendas. He talked with them instead of to them.

There was a knock on the door and Michael looked up. "Come in."

"Mike have you got a few minutes?" Natalie didn't wait for an answer and ushered in a woman who looked like she might be in her mid-30s. She held by one hand a boy who looked to be around 13 or 14 years old. "This is Susan Bishop and her son Randy. She heard your speech this morning and would like to talk to you." Natalie gave him a nod as if to mean, it's important.

"Of course." He gestured at the two chairs by his desk. "It's nice to meet you, please sit." The woman looked at him and what was on her face made him search his memory to try and recall where he'd seen that look before. "How can I help you, Ms. Bishop?"

She patted her son's hand. "Sit back Randy." The boy took out his cell phone and started playing Candy Crush. "Mr. Wharton, I listened to you this morning and for the first time I felt I was hearing from someone who knew what life was like for people like me." She glanced at her son and then back to Michael. "I'm a single mother and I've raised Randy by myself since he was a year old when my husband died. I work hard Mr. Wharton."

Michael held his hand up. "Please call me Michael."

The woman smiled almost shyly. "I work hard and in my job I'm as good as any of the men but I make less and that's wrong. And every year things are more expensive and what I do make doesn't go as far." She looked again at her son. "In five years he'll graduate from high school. He's a good kid. Gets good grades. But probably not the kind that will get him a scholarship and I'll never be able to afford to send him to college. I have had friends and family already go through this. Their kids, my nieces, and nephews... they all got student loans that'll take them years, maybe even decades, to pay off. They all got jobs though it took some of them a long time to find one." She shook her head and looked at her son again. "The jobs they found aren't high-paying. They barely get by." She looked back at Michael with her tired, worn, face already showing deep lines.

He recognized that look. That face. It was his mother's. "Ms. Bishop, I do know what it's like. And I think I know how you feel because I lived through it watching my mother raise me and it was all on her despite the fact that I did have a father. So what you've done." Michael looked at Randy who was still head down and into his cell phone game. "What you're doing for your son by caring so much. It's so much harder. And I share your concerns about equal pay, about affordable education and job opportunities that allow those who are willing to work to make a good living and not just subsist at the poverty level. I promise you — and you can find me if I don't live up to it and call me a liar to my face — that if I'm elected I will change things. I will help people turn their lives around. I will..."

Michael paused to wipe his eyes thinking about his mother's last words. "I will make things better for people like you and your son."

* * *

THE DENVER PRESS CLUB
DENVER, COLORADO

The building capacity was 230 people and it looked like there were twice that many. Michael stepped up to the dais and adjusted the microphone. "Thanks for being here with me on this beautiful spring evening," he paused glancing once at Natalie sitting in the front row. Erin Watson was sitting with her. "I believe that a leader cannot lead others until they are able to lead themselves. I know what it's like to fail at that—at leading yourself. At best your life becomes a near vacuum where you fight for each breath... at worst it's an ever tightening straightjacket, cinching tighter as get older.

"It's been pointed out that I am a relatively, young man. That's true. It's been said that I do not have any political experience. That's true, too. There are those who ask, without experience how effective can he be? They question my ability. They question whether I can get done what needs to be done.

"My answer to those questions and concerns is this:

"The American people have routinely elected experienced politicians, experienced business people, experienced military veterans. Some have worked out better than others. But look at where we are at now and where we seem to be headed. Can you say that their experience is accomplishing what you want to be done?

"For the most part, I don't think so.

"My experience in life is very different than my opponent and those behind him who are the real opposition. Instead of a motorcade, to events, including this one, I drive an old VW Beetle, several years old. At times, when its broke down I've had to push it to the side of the road—hoping I would be able to fix it or could scrape enough money together to get it fixed. I've had to decide to eat soup or what was cheap so I could pay to get a new timing belt installed. Instead of an expensive, palatial, home, I live in a cheap apartment. When I travel, I don't fly first class or get around in a chauffeured limousine. I fly coach and drive myself in a used car. I'm like most of you, one of the average citizens that make up our communities, cities, states and country.

"So my life has not been lived like those you typically elect to public office. But it has been magical. To begin with, I discovered the warmth and sense of community that comes from being with the people and not above them. In the hardest times, theirs is a feeling of hopefulness even in the face of great difficulty. I discovered the beauty of America, a vision that haunts you with its promise and potential. And most importantly for me, in living my life as I have—especially in the last two or three years—I discovered how life can be; how life should be lived. There is a universal law that if we follow can change your life. That knowledge changed mine and I've shared that particular discovery with others, some of whom call them members of my World Club. I think it's because of the people I have touched, in such a brief time, that are the reason why I am here, right now, giving this speech.

"I've been told that most people accept the perception of the value they can convince themselves of," taking a sip of water from the bottle next to the microphone. "It makes me think of Jean Moliere's statement, Things are only worth what you make them worth.

Detaching the microphone from the stand, Michael stepped from behind the podium. "I think some current events are worth talking about. Especially regarding their value—the value of human life.

"The problem of violence in America goes far beyond the issue of gun control. in actuality, when removed from a broader discussion about violence in the United States; it deflects the most significant questions that need to be raised.

"Violence saturates our culture both domestically and in our approach to foreign policy. Domestically, violence weaves through the culture like a highly charged electric current burning everything in its path. Popular culture, extending from Hollywood films and sports to video games, embraces the spectacle of violence as the primary medium of entertainment. Brutal masculine authority and the celebration of violence it embraces have become the new norm. Something we should all be concerned about in America.

"Representations of violence dominate the media and often parade before viewers as a for-profit spectacle, just as the language of violence now shapes our political discourse.

"Violence in the United States is a commodity mined for profit. An example of this would be the For-Profit Prison Industry. Violence and that the media thrives on it is a practice that has become normalized. It is a spectacle that extends the limits of the pleasure quotient in ways that should be labeled as both pathological and dangerous. We are not just voyeurs to such horrors; we have become complicit and reliant on violence as a mediating force that increasingly shapes our daily experiences. The culture of violence makes it increasingly difficult to imagine pleasure in any other terms except through the relentless spectacle of gratuitous violence and cruelty, even as we mourn its tragic effects in everyday life when it emerges in horrifying ways such as the senseless killing in Tucson, Aurora, Newtown, Charleston and San Bernardino. And we have the single deaths in Staten Island, Ferguson, Baltimore and others."

He stopped to scan the crowd, his eyes lingering longest on the reporters and media crews closest to him. "What can we do to make it stop? More laws. More guns. More police. Or is it tighter gun control laws and fewer guns and ensuring that police departments respect all citizens regardless of creed or color. All of that has been proposed and talked about in a loop of discussion that seems to have no end—and no answers." He paused long enough for the crowd to shift uncomfortably. "I know I have an answer to many of society's problems. It's old-school and harkens back to years past when more accountability was placed on the individual and less on expecting some organization or government to do the thinking and heavy lifting for us. And when I begin to talk about it... it's likely not going to be popular. Because it's hard at the individual level. The solutions to our problems all start there."

"I recently heard Erin Watson speak on the importance of teaching the subjects of Logic and Rational Thought in our schools. Nothing calls for that more than what I just said to you... the gratuitous violence and cruelty we see and hear about every day. Most are acts of irrational thought and behavior—no consideration of the consequences for others and for their self. I believe in what Erin advocates and you should, too.

"We must stop talking about doing something and start doing it. When elected I will present such a compelling rationale that I'll get others to agree, too, and start bringing to bear the tremendous power of doing what's right for the people: the children, the parents, the grandparents... for all Americans."

Behind Michael, a screen lowered and he picked up the controller from the top of the podium.

"In the package of material that you have — and if you missed getting it when you came in please let us know — you're going to read about something that some of you have already heard me talk about and some of you possibly even have experienced it from working with me." The screen lit up. "In the material and in my discussions I've talked about The Universal Law of Efficiency, I call it the ULE. Now it's something that is a certain is the law of gravity. I know you've heard of that but I doubt that you heard much beyond what I've shared with you about what following principles such as the ULE can do for you."

He pressed the button on the controller and a video began. He pressed another button to pause it. "These are YouTube videos of TED talks. The first one you'll watch this from Jeffrey Brown and the topic is how they cut youth violence in Boston by 79%. The second is from someone I know you recognize. Former Pres. Jimmy Carter. And in it he talks about why he believes the mistreatment of women is the number one human rights abuse. Now, you probably wonder what that means in regards to what I've talked about and specifically about the philosophy and principles I've developed. These two talks show a real-world application of the ULE only it hasn't been defined as such." He pressed play. "You step aside while we watch and listen." He moved away from the podium and sat in a chair at the edge of the stage.

The last video ended and he pressed stop. "In the material I gave you are links to those TED talks and to other, already in use, real-world applications of the principles behind ULE. And in each of them you can see for yourself the positive results. Now, I'm running for political office and that may be confusing, to you, as to what that means with what I'm saying about ULE. Here's how I tie the two together. I know for certain that if we lead — and to bring about change we have to do it from a broad-based government supported effort — it must be by showing that what we are proposing works at the individual level and that you're not just talking and promising in order to get elected. I am a living example of making changes at the individual level that have entirely changed my mind and my body.

And when you make those kinds of positive changes in your life it has a ripple effect that can touch and improve the lives of others. I think that if we approach government in that same way that it can solve many of the problems we face. Will no longer just kick the problems and issues down the road for someone else to face. Will hold ourselves accountable and do the right thing. The right thing for each of us as individuals and the right thing for us as a country. Thank you for being with me today and thank you for listening."

He turned from the microphone, went off stage and down the steps to where Natalie and Erin Watson were waiting for him. He took Natalie's hand, kissed her on the cheek and turned to Erin. "I didn't expect you; it's a pleasant surprise to see you again!"

She shook his hand. "Natalie called to tell me what was going on with you. I remembered our conversation that, after my talk, and was impressed with you." She smiled at Natalie and turned back to him. "I wanted to return the favor and wondered if you have time to talk?"

* * *

LATE THAT NIGHT
ERIN WATSON'S OFFICE

"I just met with him. I think you need to come see this young man speak—see how he's reaching people and how they are connecting with him. I've not seen this kind of response from anyone running for office... at least not in the last twenty or thirty years." She wrote something on the pad by the desk. "Okay... I'll send you a link to some of his writing and the transcript of some of his speeches. And his website. Let me know, okay?" Erin Watson hung up the phone.

* * *

1 AUGUST 2016
KBXS STUDIOS
DENVER, COLORADO

"Is this your first TV interview?" Caren Hunt asked as she sat in the chair on the set and motioned him to sit in the chair opposite her with a small table between.

"Yes," he replied fumbling a bit with attaching the microphone to his shirt.

"Nervous?" she smiled to put him at ease.

"A little bit," he took a sip from the bottle of water she had handed him when he sat down.

"Don't worry; I'll go easy on you," she smiled again. He wondered at how smooth and practiced that smile seemed. Knowing her and this network's reputation he questioned its genuineness. Claiming to be legitimate news what they said and covered, once passed through their filter or lens, was often mostly opinion trotted out as facts. All designed and delivered to an audience that rarely fact-checked—they took what they said as gospel. She—and this interview—would not be easy.

A man stepped over and said, "One minute to air." Michael blinked and it was on.

"This is Caren Hunt, KBXS News. I'm sitting with Michael Wharton, who is an independent candidate running against incumbent Senator Carter Blaine in the upcoming election for U.S. Senate. He has a unique platform he's running on—one not seen or heard before from a candidate for public office—that has generated a lot of buzz. We, and probably you, want to learn more about it." She paused, turned her head to face Michael and said, "Welcome, Mr. Wharton."

"Thank you for inviting me, Caren. Please call me Michael."

"Okay, so Michael, tell us why you're running for office and what you stand for—what's your message to the people and what do you offer that's so different."

"Caren, it's actually quite simple and fits well, into the seven or eight minutes you said we'd have."

He shifted to more comfortably face the camera. "It's not news that we have many issues and problems to confront; not only in Colorado but nationwide—I'd also add globally but want to stick closer to home for now. Some of these issues and problems are so big we can't come to grips with them or we believe that to resolve them requires a complex solution."

"What problems or issues are you referring to, Michael?"

"There are many, but two I've spoken about and will speak more on are inequality and the widening gap between the Haves and the Have Nots and the need to teach people—starting with the young—how to think logically and rationally."

"Two unrelated things!"

"Not really. They are related and the latter actually applies to many things we need to—and can—correct." He paused, "If we are sincere in our intent to fix them."

"You don't believe that—our politicians—your opponent wants to solve the problems we face?"

"I think most do. But I also believe they have their own reasons for the solutions they propose or for their lack of action or inattention in finding the right solution. And I believe that Senator Blaine wants to do what's right for his constituents but that belief has been filtered by a party agenda and what its advisors tell him that meet the party's backer's agenda."

"You sound like a conspiracy theorist. Surely you don't think your opponent is working against the people he represents. He's served his constituents for nearly twenty years, while you've, frankly, not done much that we can tell."

Not rising to the barbed bait, Michael continued, "Caren, most people, including politicians and my opponent, think we either need complex solutions or that the problem is just too hard to fix. We throw our hands in the air and kick the can on down the road for someone else to deal with it."

"That strikes me as a naïve perception," she said.

"It's not. Not at all. What I'm saying is that if you take individual or special interest agendas out of the equation and focus on doing what is right for the people then you can come up with simple solutions. The media, this network being particularly adept at it, makes the public fear simple solutions. It's better to keep things complicated with many convoluted moving parts. Then it's harder to see what is really going on and easier to pretend that something or someone else is the reason why things don't work as they should."

"And you can fix this. That's the reason why you're running for office."

"My reason for running for office is simple. I believe that each of us needs to learn how to resolve our inner issues so that we can hear or see clearly what the problems are and how they can be solved. We need to free ourselves from forming our thinking based on someone or some organization's opinion. An opinion crafted to serve the purpose of that organization or person's interests and not necessarily that of the public."

"You claim you've discovered some theory that can liberate people. What do you mean and I guess you must know some don't take this and you very seriously."

"It's not just a theory and I've never used the word liberate. It's about how you can change yourself so your body and mind operations more efficiently. What I've found and learned to do is as real as gravity. Some very intelligent people, doctors and scientists with the highest reputations, have seen it, not only on paper but its practical application. They believe it. I invite you and any of your viewers to find out more. It can and will make a difference in your life. And once a person has resolved those individual issues it does affect how we perceive our life and the world around us. It brings clarity to our thinking."

"Michael, with that interesting statement, we have to close." Not giving him a chance for a reply, she stood and walked toward the camera, "There's what candidate Michael Wharton believes." Shaking her head for the camera, "We all must still wonder what he's really about and how he would be a better senator than Carter Blaine for this great state and Coloradans. This is Caren Hunt for KBXS News... I'll see you tonight at 6:00 PM."

The camera light went out and she turned to Michael. Still shaking her head at him she walked past and exited stage left.

* * *

**THE WHITE HOUSE
WASHINGTON DC**

He stopped the video clip and clicked off the flat screen display and spun his chair around. Through the window could be seen the Washington Monument lighted at night. His eyes swept past it and was pleasantly surprised that he could still be moved by the sight. He reached for the phone on his credenza pressing a button. "Boss, can I come up and talk to you about something... someone I think you need to know about. Thanks, I'll be right there." Standing, he looked out the window onto the night, beyond the fence and patrolling guards. He put his jacket on and straightened his tie as he left the office. He passed his boss's oddly positioned and shaped office, on the right, as he headed to the walkway to the residence.

* * *

**CARL ROSS'S OFFICE – L STREET NW
WASHINGTON DC**

Carl Ross rarely raised his voice. He was so firmly entrenched in the bedrock of far right conservative circles he didn't need to. He was the only access to the kind of deep pockets that can swing elections. And he could deliver candidates to the owners of those pockets that would follow their agenda. He was on the phone with the Forche brothers, his deepest pockets.

"Bill, turn that thing up I can't hear Carl." Fred was five minutes older than his twin who was clearly the one really in charge. Carl heard fingers fumbling with the conference call speaker.

"Carl!" Fred's voice pitched higher.

"I'm here Fred." He leaned toward the microphone and the base of his own office system.

"So, you going to take care of this boy?" The clunk clunk sound told Carl that Fred had put his size 16 cowboy boots on the table. "The one that's giving Blaine so much trouble."

"Yes, Fred. My media director is ready."

"Well, I want you to really drag this kid through the dirt."

"Carter's not keen on that. He wants to deal just with issues."

"That won't work." It was Bill's quiet even tone that was such a contrast to Fred's bluster. "We need the people to feel alarmed that this young man would be the wrong choice. His election would put their freedom... their livelihood at risk."

"We can't make him seem to have Muslim ties, can we?" Fred asked.

"No, Fred. He's white, born and raised in Colorado, a Christian though not affiliated. He's not done much of anything wrong or right with his life. Nothing. He was pretty ordinary until about a year ago."

"How are you going to spin him then?" The rasping, dragging, sound meant the boots were off the table.

"He has some clearly defined beliefs that he feels are responsible for turning his life around."

"How the hell does that-"

A louder voice overrode him. Bill must've moved closer. "I don't understand. How can that be used?"

Carl opened a dossier folder on the table in front of him. "It's an unusual philosophy. Let me give you an overview and how we plan to attack him."

* * *

COMMUNITY COLLEGE OF DENVER, CONFLUENCE BUILDING DENVER, COLORADO

"Bob Allen, CBS News: Mr. Wharton, why don't you have a spokesperson or press secretary?"

"There are too many opportunities to use one to play word games with the media and with the public. When you want an answer to a question, you'll get it direct from me. When you want to know what I think about a topic. You'll get it from me. No adulteration or filter. Life is not scripted and decisions are not made in a perfect world where things are rehearsed and staged. I'm not perfect so no doubt may say things that some people take exception to but in any and all decisions for the public interest they will receive proper deliberation and well-reasoned judgment."

"Carl Ross, Senator Blaine's top advisor, claims your way of thinking would jeopardize our national security," said Caren Hunt as she stuck her microphone under his nose.

"Mr. Ross is entitled to his opinion, as inaccurate as it may be," Michael replied then paused to give her a chance and any others that wanted to continue the line of the question.

She kept it going. "Is it true that you and he had some harsh words backstage before tonight's event? The word is you hate each other intensely because of your respective views."

"That's not true. I don't dislike anyone because of their opinions—I respect that everyone has a right to their own," Michael paused long enough for the crowd chatter to quiet down then spoke loudly. "I don't like Carl Ross because he sucks as a human being. The unfortunate thing is that he grooms political candidate that appear to be on the side of the people but, in fact, are not—they have an agenda. And it's Carl Ross's."

"Aren't you concerned that statement will be viewed as a personal attack? Shouldn't politics be above taking things to a personal level?"

"Your question assumes that politicians or their advisors and handlers should not be judged based on who they are as people—as individuals. But where do character and integrity come from if not the individual?"

"You didn't answer my question. Are you worried about repercussions when you make a statement like that? "

"No. I'm not concerned," Michael stood silent for a moment. "I believe you have to make hard observations and tell the public how you feel about a topic... or a person; if that person factors into the public discourse and decision making of an elected official. I'm not a saint or a perfect man. My flaws and issues are out there for all to dissect. I'm okay with that and made a conscious decision to change my life from what was to what I want it to be. Many believe that what I've done and believe in can benefit others. To reach the broadest group of people with the greatest potential to bring about positive change is why I decided to run for office. And when I made that decision I knew I could only do it one way. I would answer questions directly, not be disingenuous or dance around them trying to pass a lot of ambiguous words off as a response."

"That sounds great if you stick to it," said one of the correspondents in the front row.

"I will and if I don't you can call me on it," Michael replied with a smile. "Now, I have something to direct at you folks. For the most part, many in the media do not have the backbone to ask hard questions—especially of politicians or political candidates." He looked at Caren Hunt and added, "Especially if there a candidate you support—or our handlers are backing." He looked away from her and at the other reporters. "I'm not sure why the hard questions aren't pressed home to get a clear answer. Is it a sense of political—no pun intended—correctness? Is it that you're afraid of some form of backlash? Is it that you just don't care or don't want the hard work that follows when you stir the pot?" He scanned them from left to right. "The one thing I do know is that it sucks. The public expects and used to be able to rely on journalists and news reporters to ask tough questions. And to get answers or cut through the interviewee's silence or obfuscation—to show the public exactly who they are. If you can't get a straight response to a direct question, the reporter should skewer the person they are interviewing. Instead, we see verbal volleyball with no desire for points to be scored. It's just meaningless passing the ball back and forth."

He looked pointedly at Caren Hunt, who commanded a prominent position in the cluster of reporters. She smirked at him.

"I'll leave you with this because as much as you want me to shoot straight I want you, the media, to do it too. This a quote from Jon Stewart: Journalists have abandoned their responsibilities through a mix of indifference and a lack of gumption that leaves viewers and readers with no real idea of what is going on."

Michael started to turn to go and stopped. "I recently talked with a young man— that's him and his father." He pointed to the front row where an older man sat next to a younger version of himself. "Hi, Sam and Stephen. We talked about black lives but even more importantly we talked about that all lives matter. And he asked something that all of us, I believe, have asked at some time or the other. It used to be just during election time but now, since things are changed so radically, elections and politicians running campaigns to either be elected or reelected seem to last year round. It never ends." Michael shook his head. "Stephen, asked me why it is that no one in politics gives a straight answer. I told him what I'll tell you now. I swear if you ask me direct questions I will give you direct answers. If I don't have one I can give you immediately, I will say so. But I won't try to bluff my way through it."

He heard a sound like a laugh and caught Hunt leaning over saying something to another reporter. He noted that one of her aids with a handheld video camera had panned from him to her.

* * *

MICHAEL'S CAMPAIGN OFFICE

"Thanks," He told the staffer that handed him the note. He looked down at it and all it had was a phone number with area code 202. At the top of the note was written, THEY SAID IT WAS VERY IMPORTANT. Shrugging, he dialed the number.

"Hello Michael."

"Who is this?"

He heard the man chuckle. "I never cared for Caren Hunt. Her zealotry makes me think of McCarthy at his height back in the 50s."

Michael recognize the voice but couldn't place it. "I'm sorry but who is this?"

"Benjamin Hargrove."

Michael swallowed air and almost coughed. "Mr. President!"

"So they say and by the grace of the people of the United States." He chuckled. "Now, I know you're probably puzzled. Why the call?" He paused and it was quiet on the line. "You there, son?"

"Yes or · - I'm here. How can I help you, sir?"

"It seems that some people that work for me have become fans of yours. Well one of them that works for me still, my Chief of Staff, Ron Eldridge. And he got a call from someone, a lady that I have great respect for. Erin Watson. She had some great things to say about you to Ron and then to me as well."

"Thank you, sir."

"Ron is in Boulder and wants to meet with you later tonight. He's going to talk to you about some things that I have in mind. You might find them surprising given that I'm a Republican and you're an independent running against an incumbent Republican Senator. I think we're at a point, as a country, where the old rules — the old mechanisms and ways — need to be changed. Not the things that clearly work, like our Constitution. But the things that we've done to the system. I don't think it's sustainable. Not if we want our country to grow stronger and not just militarily but perhaps morally and socially so that we become a role model for the world again. Ron and Erin both have shown me videos of your speeches, your press conferences and what you're doing there in Colorado. And frankly I'm impressed. Now, I like Carter Blaine your opponent. He's a good man. But like many of us including me I admit that being a good man in a flawed system doesn't do much good for this country. I don't know about this whole ULE thing you talk about but given what I've seen so far and how you're connecting and engaging the people of Colorado I'll tell you this. If you get elected we'll talk more about how what you're doing, what you believe, may work at a national level with my support behind you. For now, here in a little while you'll get a call from Ron and he'll set up a meeting to talk with you further. Good luck son."

"Thank you si—" Michael realized the president had hung up. He didn't know what to think. He didn't know if he should tell Natalie and there was no way in hell he would tell Larry because Larry would blab it to everyone. He started to put the cell phone back in his pocket when it buzzed. He looked at it. Area code 202 but a different number. "Hello?"

CHAPTER SEVEN

"I... mark in every face I meet
Marks of weakness, marks of woe.
In every cry of every man,
In every infant's cry of fear,
In every voice, in every ban,
The mind-forged manacles I
hear..."

—William Blake

27 SEPTEMBER 2016
MICHAEL'S CAMPAIGN OFFICE

"I think they're getting desperate." Natalie said and Larry sitting next to her grinned.

Michael looked tired. It showed around the eyes and how he seemed to have to consciously sit up straight instead of slipping into the chair. "Maybe they are. They called me everything but by my right name, it seems. And they're taking shots at you guys, too."

Larry's grin got even bigger. "I can take it. They can call me a coffee serving slacker all they want."

Michael looked at Natalie. "And they branded you as a traitor."

"What they say or think doesn't matter. It just shows they will throw a label on someone and if they can make it stick — that I'm the treasonous spoiled yet dissatisfied daughter of Carter Blaine — then it serves their purpose. But only if I let it get to me. And it doesn't because it's not true. My father has told them so and even told them to back off. But they won't. It's can escalate like this until the election and maybe even afterward." She sighed. "I've seen this happen with my father's campaigns, but it's a lot different when you're on the other side of it."

Michael walked to the corkboard with the campaign calendar pin to it. It was a long-term plan or that now had most of the days' boxes crossed out. "At first I didn't like your father Natalie but I've come to respect him. I see in him what you told me that he used to be like when he was younger." He turned and came back to the couch to sit next to me. He took her hand and held it in both of his. "If I'm elected and in 10 or fifteen years if I'm still in office, will I end up like him?"

Natalie leaned over, kissed him, and rested her head on his shoulder. "Michael you don't understand or maybe you do and just won't say it. You are and you're not like my father. You have some of his good qualities but none of the bad. Maybe that's the ULE at work in you but also I think it's because you're going into this with blinders completely off. You know what's wrong and you have a plan for how to fix it. I think when you go into it that way it's not able to twist you and change you as it did my father. Even now, in your debates with my father and all the discussions when he's talking to you he seems younger and more like the man he was during his first term. For that…" She kissed him again. "I think you. You've given me that side of my father back."

"Well, you two…" He looked at Natalie and then Larry. "I don't think they can get any worse; there's not much else they can do except call us more bad names."

* * *

THAT EVENING
27 SEPTEMBER 2016

"Only for a friend," muttered Larry, not really mad but not pleased he had to dash across the street in a downpour to get the car for Michael and Natalie. The slick pavement was bad enough wearing men's dress shoes much less Natalie's high-heels. At least Mike had given him his overcoat and hat to help keep off the rain while he continued to press the flesh with some of the rich ladies backing his campaign. Natalie held her umbrella over him at the curb waiting for traffic to clear so he could make his dash. Just down the sidewalk, near where the entrance to and exit from the parking garage met the street, was a string of news vans. Each with a satellite dish and a morose looking driver sitting behind the wheel or standing on the sidewalk as if watching or waiting for something or someone.

Further down the street a gray sedan sat idling. Seeing Natalie with a man at the curb the driver stubbed out the cigarette and clicked his seatbelt in place. As Larry stepped off the curb, the driver dropped the car in gear and surged forward, car lights out and hard to see in the rain darkened twilight. Larry was almost at the concrete median when the car hit him. His body flipped over the hood, sliding up the windshield and off to the side. On the impact, he felt the snapping of his legs and then nothing more when his head struck the concrete. The car kept accelerating, running the red light and was soon out of sight.

* * *

28 SEPTEMBER 2016
RALLY FOR MICHAEL WHARTON
BOULDER, COLORADO

"My friend, Larry, died last night. He died because he believed in me—helped me—was always there for me. He was in the wrong place at the wrong time because of me." Michael paused, his hands at his side tightening to a white knuckled clench, but there was nothing for them to grip.

"Larry also believed that the United States is the greatest nation in the world to live. It welcomed his mother and gave her a chance she would never have had in her home country. The opportunity to work hard... to work two and sometimes three jobs just to get by and eventually to set enough money aside to start her own small business. And by continuing to work hard she saw that her son had good clothes and a decent education I believe America is a great country, too. But we have problems. The truth is, in so many ways of measurement; in so many critical areas like education, life expectancy, income and other metrics; the U.S. no longer leads the world. But we could again... if we admit the truth of where things stand and work to fix the problems that have created a downward slide. In Shakespeare's Julius Caesar, Cassius was right: The fault, dear Brutus, is not in our stars, but in ourselves. Another quote, this one from Edward R. Murrow, is a fundamental reason why we, and the politicians we elect, struggle with solving our nation's problems: A great many people think they are thinking when they are merely rearranging their prejudices.

"You want to help our country become the leader it can be again?

"Stop prejudice. Look at the example we set the world with events, unwarranted violence against black people.

"Stop the mindless following.

"Stop accepting it when the media, or politicians, or whoever, blows smoke up the collective ass of the American public (or your ass individually) to make them (or you) believe something that is not true. Just so they can get the ratings or get elected or benefit in some way from that happening.

"Stop the ridiculous notion that those who point out the problems we have as a nation are unpatriotic and don't love their country. That's bullshit. Those who believe we don't love our country, in fact, are part of the problem. They are simple minded, hidebound individuals who do not think—they merely rearrange their prejudices letting others do their thinking for them – or they have their own agenda which they will benefit from by making statements that it's unpatriotic to say we are no longer the leader of the world in many ways. As an example, we live in what we feel is the best country in the world. But statistics show a different picture of Americans when compared to citizens of countries that spend much less on healthcare and have much less sophisticated infrastructure, including medical technology. Thirty-five years ago, babies born in the U.S. had an infant mortality rate equal to Germany. Today, American babies die at twice the rate of those in Germany. Thirty-five years ago, the U.S. ranked 13th in life expectancy for girls among the thirty-four recognized industrial societies. Today we are ranked 29th out of those same thirty-four countries. We have the highest teenage birth rate in the industrialized world. One out of every four children in this country lives with a single parent, the highest rate by far in the industrialized world. A separate topic and one I've mentioned previously about the For-Profit Prison Industry. Our incarceration rate is triple what it was four decades ago, with an incarceration rate five times that of other wealthy democracies. Why is that? Is it that our citizens are so much worse than theirs? I don't think so, but we need to find the answer. And it's you, the individual, that can help most in getting them from your elected officials.

"Start to face facts—if you don't have them—demand them.

"Start to think for yourself.

"Political ads are designed to play on fears. Are intended to shackle clear thinking. Are designed to make the viewer "a simple button to push."

"Push enough and get elected.

"The people don't want ads and TV commercials like that. The people deserve, and should demand, better. The people—the working class people that make up the majority of Americans—just want politicians that do their jobs and that are proper stewards of our trust. And that they serve the interest of the people.

"Not just at the beginning.

"Not just enough to get elected.

"Not just while everyone is looking or listening.

"They want leaders to feel that responsibility deep inside—for now—for tomorrow—for always (or at least as long as they are in office).

"I see the rallies and I see those not on such a stage. I understand the needs of the people.

"I'll leave you with this one question you should ask yourself: once the elections are over... will I see the leaders we so sorely need? I hope you, those listening, chose to vote for the person who comes closest to the ideal of working with facts and on issues, not distortions, fear, and trading insults.

"That must be your criteria. That is the person who should get your vote."

* * *

29 SEPTEMBER 2016
SENATOR CARTER BLAINE'S OFFICE

Carter Blaine slammed the door, "What the hell are you doing?" he turned to face Carl Ross, who had taken a seat and looked up, imperturbably, at him.

"Doing?"

"You know what I mean. If you or any of your people had anything to do with last night..."

"You're slipping in the polls," Ross interrupted. "That's not good. Your backers are... concerned.

"That boy..."

"Died in a tragic accident. Very sad," he shrugged. "But hit and runs do occur, don't they?"

Ross stood walked to the door, pausing before opening it he turned to look at Blaine, "Accidents happen, sometimes to those we love."

The door clicked shut and Blaine sat silently for a moment. A quarter turn and he reached for the framed photograph. Her eyes looked into his—they had been so full of life—they had been so young. She had always been able to communicate with him by a gesture, an uplifted eyebrow or merely the sparkle in her eyes. He now saw, in her eyes, the reflection of his own questions about how his life had turned out.

* * *

21 OCTOBER 2016
THE BLAINE RESIDENCE

"What do you mean back off? Quit? Michael should just hand the election to you? Well not to you but to those guys that own you!" Natalie was white-faced with anger.

The gray hair that once only peppered temples was now shot throughout his hair. Carter Blaine swept it back with his hand. "I'm sorry about Michael's friend. But-"

"He was my friend too!" she cried.

"I know, Natalie... I know. And I'm sorry about his accident." He tried to put his arm around her shoulders. She shrugged him off and headed to the door.

"Does getting elected mean that much to you?" she snapped.

He walked toward her his hands out trying to placate her. "Honey, this isn't about the election. It's about us — what's driven us apart. The elections not as important as fixing what I've broken. Rebuilding what I've lost and regaining your trust in me."

"Dad, I love you but you set your goons on Michael and now Larry is dead. I don't know if I can forgive you. I don't care if Michael loses the election. Because he won't have lost me. But you have." She slammed the door behind her.

He stood staring at the back of the door for a long moment. He walked to the mirror over the table that ran along the wall. He looked at his reflection. He wondered about the man in the mirror and what had happened to him. That man he had been to his little girl so many years ago. He went to his desk and sat down. Picking up the folder showing the results from the latest polls he wondered if he'd ever look in the mirror and find him there. Would she ever see him like that again?

* * *

28 OCTOBER 2016
MICHAEL'S APARTMENT

He turned the television off. He couldn't take any more of the news and the endless repeating of the circumstances behind Larry's death; the campaign and election coverage and everything else going on in the world. "Natalie?"

"Yes," she called from the kitchen.

He went to her. "This election — if I lose it's not the end of the world. I can still teach people about the ULE. Just like I was doing before all of this." Michael waved his arms around encompassing the room, the apartment building, the city. "Everything."

"I know. It's not what happens to us that defines us." She gave him a hug. "Hand me those dishes." She took them from him rinsing them in the sink and placing in the dishwasher. She straightened drying her hands on a kitchen towel. "It's what we do after something happens to us that counts. Right?" She winked at him as she poured two glasses of tea and then handed one to him. "That straight from that book Indira gave you."

Michael laughed and followed her into the living room. "I see you've been reading." She moved one of the cushions to make room for to sit next to her. He raised his glass and she cleaned hers against it. "No matter what we're together and that's what counts."

CHAPTER EIGHT

"If you can bear to hear the truth, you've spoken. Twisted by knaves to make a trap for fools. Or watch the things you gave your life to, broken. And stoop and build them up with worn-out tools…"
—Rudyard Kipling, IF

8 NOVEMBER 2016, ELECTION NIGHT
CARTER BLAINE'S CAMPAIGN HEADQUARTERS

The results did not look promising—anything but—the numbers were running against him. Carter Blaine stood, and told his handlers and hangers-on, he needed a moment as he stepped into another room of the suite. He sat at the room's desk and using a piece of stationery wrote for several minutes filling the sheet without pause. Done, he stared at what he had written but not seeming to look at the words. He put the note in an envelope and carefully wrote a name on it. Standing up he stepped over and opened the door into the sitting area—the group of people still staring at the television as if mesmerized. Walking across to the entrance, he caught one of his staffer's eye, and with a come-here nod, handed him the envelope, "I want you to hand-deliver this; go now but don't hand it over until things are final."

Stepping back into the room he walked over to Carl Ross and leaned over, "We need to talk... privately... outside." Ross looked at him with a mixture of questioning and irritation but followed him out the door of the room. Walking over to the elevators Blaine quieted Ross with a gesture. Taking the elevator down to the parking garage they walked over to the black Mercedes in the VIP parking spot.

"Get in Carl... Don't ask questions just get in."

"What the hell are you doing Carter? In about 30 minutes, you're going to have to give a concession speech and I have to start doing some major damage control. So I repeat. What in the hell are we doing here?"

Carter was a large man and still in shape. He took Ross's arm and led him to the car and opened it for him. "Get in Carl." There was a handful of people also going to their cars. A couple of them stopped, recognizing the senator they took out their cell phones and started taking pictures. "I don't think it would serve either of our interests if this turns into a confrontation. Do you?"

Carl sneered, "Reverting to type aren't you—the hot-headed poor kid from the streets?" The look on Blaine's face didn't change, but his grip intensified. Wincing he got in.

Outside the parking garage the rain was coming down harder with the slushy weight of ice. Pulling on the highway it was thick with traffic into the city and beyond leaving the Westin he turned left on Lawrence and then right on Speer then onto I25. The street lights shone wetly as the limo accelerated from the city center.

* * *

BREAKING NEWS: Senator Carter Blaine has been involved in a traffic accident. The Senator had evidently left the Westin downtown just before the election was called for his opponent Michael Wharton. Facing a concession speech that would no doubt have been unpleasant to give it's not known why the Senator along with his advisor Carl Ross left the hotel. Both men were apparently not wearing seatbelts and were found injured when police and paramedics arrived at the scene. They've been taken to BCH Trauma Center.

CHAPTER NINE

It was early morning. White-faced, still wearing the dress from the previous evening, Natalie met an arc of reporters with Michael at her side. He stepped up to the dais.

"This morning is tough, especially for my fiancée, Natalie. You've all heard about the accident her father was involved in. Natalie was with him at the hospital until a short while ago and reports that he is in ICU but stable. We pray for his speedy recover. Once I'm done here Natalie and I will head to BCH to be with him.

"I did not agree with Senator Blaine on many things and I do not mean any disrespect when I say I feel he was a good man that got lost somewhere along the way in his life... especially his political life. Being good and then slipping from what made you that way does not make you a contradiction as a person. It means you are a human who went sideways—that happens in life. It probably happens to more people than most would admit. We cut ourselves, or our set of morals, short. We look for the expedient... the quick reward because many don't want to do what is necessary to build what is right. That's true for individuals and I think it is true for societies and countries. So we have some illogic... some incongruence that creeps into our life and into our politics.

"In many ways, my family's life... my life... reflects some of the contradictions of America, and indeed, Americans as a whole. The history of America is one of striving for independence. It is the story of people fighting to be free from the rule of a monarchy; A story of the leadership of not only of great men like Lincoln and Washington but also ordinary people who endured great hardship, to secure self-determination in the face of great odds.

"But for all the progress that has been made. We must surely acknowledge that many Americans have yet to fulfill their potential. That the hopefulness many used to feel, because of failures in corporate and political leadership has been replaced by cynicism and sometimes despair. And that real freedom has not yet been won for those struggling to live day to day, week to week or month to month. Ordinary citizens who continue to find themselves trapped in the crossfire of political rhetoric and hyperbole—between words and lip service are angry. They need their concerns addressed. They elect politician they think will help them. Only to see them lie to become elected, follow the agenda of the powerful so they can remain in office... with little thought of serving the people that voted them into that office.

"Statistics powerfully describe this unfulfilled promise. More people struggle paycheck-to-paycheck than ever before. Unemployment levels, while improving, are still a primary concern and yet anyone looking at our decaying infrastructure can see that there is much to be done in America.

"How can we explain this fact? Certainly it is not due to lack of effort on the part of ordinary Americans. We know how hard Americans are willing to work, the tremendous sacrifices that parents make for their children, the Herculean efforts they make for their families. We know equally well the talent, the intelligence, and the creativity that exists in this country. And we know how much this land is blessed— with great gifts and riches. Yet we have a widening gap in incomes. The rich are richer, the middle class is shrinking, slipping in a direction that belies the American dream most of us were raised believing in. And the poor are trapped and many will likely never climb out of the hole they are in.

"We have a political system with a history of outside influences that explains why politics has become so polarizing. We have failed, to some degree, to create a government that is transparent and accountable. One that serves its people and is free from special interest groups and those who have a personal agenda.

"There is no doubt that what Americans have accomplished throughout its history is both impressive and inspiring. Among the world's nations, America remains a model for representative democracy—a place where many different ethnic factions have found a way to live and work together in peace and stability. We enjoy a robust civil society; a press—media—that's, for the most part, free, fair, and honest.

"And yet, the reason I speak of the freedoms we have is because today it is in jeopardy. It is being threatened by those who want the public to think one way—theirs. That's not a new problem. It's a human problem, and it has existed in some form in almost every society. From patronage machines to questionable elections. In just the last few years, our own U.S. Congress has seen a representative resign after taking bribes, and several others fall under investigation for using their public office for private gain.

"But while this is a problem we all share; it is a crisis that's robbing an honest people of the opportunities they have fought for—the chance they deserve.

"I know that while recent reports have pointed to returned economic growth in this country, too many still live in poverty. And I know that the vast majority of people in this country desperately want to change this.

"It is painfully evident that the old ways of thinking stifles development—and political self-interest siphons off scarce resources that could improve infrastructure, bolster education systems, and strengthen public health. It stacks the deck so high against entrepreneurs that they cannot get their job-creating ideas off the ground. It erodes the state from the inside out, sickening the justice system until there is no truth to be found, poisoning the police forces until their presence becomes a source of insecurity rather than comfort.

"Stress has a way of magnifying the very worst inside us and makes even worse the adverse twists of fate. It makes it impossible to respond adequately to crises -- whether it's an economic meltdown, flu pandemic or crippling drought.

"The flaws in our system and in some people's perceptions can also provide opportunities for those who would harness the fear and hatred of others to their agenda and ambitions.

"It can shield them from being asked the hard questions and to provide legitimate answers.

"Some of the worst actors also take advantage of the collective exhaustion and outrage that people feel and with that comes a new set of distortions and betrayals of public trust.

"In the end, if the people cannot trust their government to do the job for which it exists—to protect them and to promote their common welfare—all else is lost. And this is why the struggle against what constricts us is one of the great struggles of our time.

"The good news is that there are already signs of progress. Willingness to apply new thinking is increasingly significantly. Some of the people that I've worked with over the past couple of years have been courageous in taking the steps necessary to change their own lives. During my campaign, in uncovering and reporting on some of the most blatant abuses of the system, there has been growing recognition among people and politicians that this is a critical issue.

"The renewed vigor in the belief that we as an individual can improve. That as a society and country we can change what is wrong and build on what is right means a promising future for all Americans.

"This election is one of the steps taken to fulfill the promise. But elections are not enough. In a genuine democracy, it is what happens between elections that are the true measure of how great that country really is or can become.

"Today, we're starting to see that people want more than a mere changing of the guard, more than piecemeal reforms and bandages slapped on to attempt to cure what is crippling their country. The people are crying out for real change. And so we know that there is more work to be done—more reforms to be made. I don't have all the solutions or think that they'll be easy, but there are a few places that a country truly committed to reform could start.

"Finally, fear-based politics has to stop. It is rooted in the bankrupt idea that the goal of politics or business is to funnel as much of the pie as possible to one's own pocket, political, organization or commercial for-profit circle with little regard for the public good. It stifles innovation and fractures the fabric of the society. Instead of opening businesses and engaging in commerce, people come to rely on patronage and payback as a means of advancing. Instead of unifying the country to move forward in solving problems, it divides neighbor from neighbor.

"An accountable, transparent government can break this cycle. When people are judged on merit, not connections, then the best and brightest can lead the country, people will work hard, and the entire economy will grow—everyone will benefit and more resources will be available for all, not just select groups.

"Of course, in the end, one of the strongest weapons our country has to fight against what is wrong is the ability of you, the people, to stand up and speak out about the injustices you see. The people are the ultimate guardians against abuses.

"By rejecting the idea that we cannot change, these heroes reveal the very opposite. They show strength and integrity of character that can make a great country even greater and build the type of future we owe generations to come in the United States. By focusing on creating strong, independent individuals rather following the cults of personality, they make a contribution to their country that will last longer than their own lives. They fight the battle of our time.

It all starts with individuals who believe in a better way. They believe in a better life and that they control how that life unfolds. It's about living life with an unlocked soul."

* * *

THAT EVENING
BCH TRAUMA CENTER – BOULDER

Natalie handed Michael the letter that the staffer had brought from her father. "What's this?"

"It's from my father. He sent it to me last night. When I read it I thought it was a copy of his concession speech and I guess in a way it was. But it was for me." She looked at her father who was still unconscious and hooked to a myriad of machines and monitors.

Seeing Carter Blaine, he thought of his mother's struggle and how she spent her last days in such a bed. "What does it say?"

"Go ahead you can read it."

He opened the envelope and took out the sheet of personal stationery. Unfolding it he leaned to the side to hold under the light:

Carter Blaine

8 November 2016

Over a long career in politics I realize now that while I've done some good I have certainly not done what I could have and should have.

Tonight, for the first time in a very long time, I tasted defeat. Though I've been proud to serve the people of Colorado for many years now. I wasn't born into life as a senator and with all the blessings, opportunities and benefits that come with such a position. But somehow, along the way and enjoying them, thanks to the good citizens of Colorado, I forgot where I came from and what I had set out to do as a young man when I first ran for office.

Over that time, operating within our political system and the way things are, I learned a great deal. I realize now that in the future if I'm ever to be truly productive and useful I need to unlearn much of it. And it's ironic that a young man, who at first I chose to patronize and feel superior to, has shown me, an older and far more experienced person, the right way to be a man... to be a human being.

So now I'm faced with acknowledging not only defeat but also that I've been wrong in many ways. You know I used to think that such a thing would be too bitter to contemplate. Losing. Admitting my flaws. But instead I feel liberated by them. Because it's only through acknowledging and admitting their fact — their existence. That I can go about the work of fixing them.

I have much work to do on myself. Here in Colorado there is much work to do for our beautiful state and its citizens. But I'll start with me and then go from there. I do plan to reach out to that young man. To Michael Wharton and offer to help him in any way that I can.

My daughter, Natalie... I'm so sorry for not remaining the type of father that I should've been for you after your mother died. I hope that you give me an opportunity to show you that there is still part of him inside me and with your love and help I can become all that you used to admire so many years ago.

CHAPTER TEN

Newton was asked how he made his discoveries. "By intending my mind on them," he replied. This steady pressure, this becoming one with what we seek to understand, whether it be atom or soul, is the one means to know. When we become a thing, we really know it, not otherwise.

FOUR YEARS LATER
SENATOR MICHAEL WHARTON'S OFFICE
WASHINGTON DC

The gray-haired man entered his office. "Thanks for taking the time to see me, Senator." The grin carried with it just a vestige of the old Carter Blaine.

"I can't tell if that's sincere or if you've been inhabited by Larry's ghost and taken the smart ass path." Michael laughed rising and coming from around his desk to shake his hand.

Carter had with him several folders and set them on the corner of Michael's desk. "Well, I guess it might be a little of both." He smiled. "May I?" He gestured at one of the plush chairs next to Michael's desk and promptly sat down. "How does it feel to win your first reelection?"

"You know what that's like." Michael nodded.

Carter looked around. "This hasn't changed much."

"Can I get you drink?" Michael waved at the side table that had an assortment of cans, cups, bottles and ice bucket.

Carter stood and walked over to the wall where a plaque was prominently displayed.

The ULE Principles

1. I will keep myself and other people safe at all times.
2. I know I have the courage to follow my highest values.
3. I choose cooperative rather than competitive actions.
4. I believe that all solutions start with the individual.
5. I accept full responsibility for my actions.
6. I am aware of and will release tension within my own body.
7. I will strive to reduce tension in all others.
8. I will reduce unnecessary resistance with my personal choices.
9. I will work to reduce unnecessary resistance worldwide to help others.

10. I will work to reduce resistance in all who I come in contact with for seven generations to come.

"I remember the first time I met you and you looked at the plaque on my wall in my study. You made some comments about them."

Michael had joined him. "I remember there were several of them that I thought were just plain wrong. I still believe that and that these are much better and go a lot further in solving problems for people."

Carter went back to the chair by the desk. "I agree with you. But mostly because they're not just words on paper or etched into a plaque on the wall. It's because I've learned to use them and it's as if I've lightened my soul. I never realized how heavy it'd been to carry around all those years."

"What's on the agenda?" Michael pointed at the folders. "Is that from the White House?"

Carter took the top folder from the stack and opened it. "This is some of the data that they've collected—most of it from the outgoing administration but some new data, too—from the statewide programs on health benefits that they're starting to see. Most of it appears to be represented by fewer emergency room visits for anxiety and stress related incidents. They expect to confirm the downturn in health costs once they get the data back from the American Medical

Association (AMA) and statewide doctor groups that are tracking data for us now. The president is pleased."

Michael leaned back in his chair. "Well, it's been a process to get in place, but starting with Colorado we managed to work our way outward state-by-state and get full implementation. I think this time next year we'll really see, certainly statistically, the benefits."

Carter open the second folder. "I've met with different congressional committees the leaders from both sides of the aisle in the Senate and House and also senior advisors in the Administration. There seems to be less infighting and more bipartisan cooperation and that's led to what might possibly be the most productive sessions in decades. I think we can say that more people in government are on board. And mostly it's because their constituents are driving that and that's how it should be. The influence of lobbyists and special interest groups are waning because collectively they just don't have the power they once had. Now, more people are taking things into their own hands and forming their own opinions based on facts. And frankly it's because they feel better."

He opened the last folder, a thin, red, one. "And now this one." He opened the last folder the thin, red, one. "The president is going to invite you to the White House to talk about you addressing the United Nations to present what the United States has accomplished so far with the ULE and how it may be used internationally."

Michael uncrossed his arms and scratched his neck. "I wonder if it's too soon. You sure the president said he wanted me to talk to the U.N.?"

"He was adamant. He's already called the Secretary-General, Margot Akerstrom of Sweden, and she'd like to arrange a private meeting with you in New York City next week. Now, that meeting wouldn't be for your speech to the General Assembly. Your meeting with her would be to present an overview of how you implemented the ULE here in the United States and the metrics... what are the measurables to judge its effectivity that they, too, could use. Once she gets a grasp of it... a date will be set for your speech."

Michael took that in. The thought of how far he'd come in such a relatively short amount of time still made him pause to reflect. "You remember when you woke up in the hospital and Natalie and I sat with you for days until you got out? We talked for hours."

"The conversations were excellent." He rubbed the scar that ran from the edge of his temple into the thick, now entirely gray, hair. "Other things about it weren't so good." He grimaced. "You know, at first when you started talking about the ULE, its principles and how they work from a practical perspective. I thought it would be a way to reduce regulatory interference with businesses and how that would be a great boost to the economy."

Michael nodded. "I argued with you that what that would do is give corporations carte blanche to maximize their bottom line by cutting costs or doing things that, in the end, were detrimental and in some cases down-right dangerous, for the public. And how that became an escalator of resistance, tension and distrust. It would be counter to everything ULE can achieve for us."

"You got me thinking straight. I admit you were right." He grew quiet. "One of the things that Natalie mentioned to me, especially early on back before you ran against me. Was the people that you had helped that actually had an illness or health issues that they struggled with that medicine treated but couldn't ever cure. Do you ever hear from them or from any of the people that have come to the ULE through the statewide and national outreach program?"

"All the time. I get updates from people back in Boulder and all over the United States." Michael turned and picked up a green folder from the credenza behind him. It was thick with papers. "Email, postcards, handwritten letters..." He looked up at Carter and smiled. "I've got Janice in St. Louis," he slid an email out. "Who wrote to tell me how well she was doing and that her multiple sclerosis no longer controlled her life." He pulled out a postcard. "Stephen Hellwig in

Boise Idaho — diabetes completely gone. And there's dozens more." He closed the folder and put it back on his credenza. "You know what I used to tell people when I would talk with them face-to-face about what was wrong with their body and how the ULE could help them? First you need to believe in the process that you're using. Part of that is the placebo effect. It's a known influence."

"You're not talking about just fooling someone into thinking they're getting better are you?" Carter looked hard at Michael.

"Not that at all. If you don't believe that the process will help you heal, then you're not going to be willing to do it and it takes time and energy. You need to want to heal. If you don't want to heal, or feel like a victim, you won't have the energy or motivation to heal. You need to have the resources to restore your health: food, water, sleep. There are certain biochemical things that the body needs to have enough energy to heal. For this to work, you need to have the time to do the meditation and it takes energy to heal. Again, a fundamental law of physics. Can't get around that. You have to be willing to do what it takes to heal. If you're not willing to say rehab after surgery, you won't heal as well. If you're not willing to stop smoking when you have lung cancer, you're not going to heal. In terms of the energy required, you have to be willing to do the hard work it takes to get in touch with the underlying reasons for the tension. For example, if someone has a lot of tension because of say, sexual abuse issues, they will have that tension for the rest of their life if they're not willing to bring that up to consciousness and let go of it. Tension is the body's mechanism for fighting against emotional experiences or issues. There've been times when I might feel like crying, but I didn't want to. So instead I tighten up so I won't feel. If I get hit physically, I will tighten up against the pain. If I get hit emotionally, I'll do the same to not experience the emotional pain or trauma. First of all, all parents program their children whether consciously or subconsciously despite best intentions. So for a child dealing with emotional issues, they take on the emotional programming of their parents. They don't open up and deal with it as they should, because the parents might not be comfortable. But for the child holding onto that is necessary resistance, because children need their parents and their connection with their parents. The point is holding onto that kind of programming is necessary for a young child, but it is not needed for an adult. We grow up and hold onto that stuff and most people can't get back in touch with letting themselves go. That tension makes the body not work efficiently, like the analogy of the engine with the bearings too tight. We as adults don't have to hold onto that tension. It is unnecessary resistance."

Carter checked an alert that popped up on his smartphone. He looked up at Michael.

"What are you smiling at? You look like the Cheshire cat." Carter had retrieved the folders and had them resting on his lap. He was staring at Michael.

"I think the big boss has something else planned for you, too."

"What?" Michael asked.

"He just got elected, too—boosted by former President Hargrove, whose second term was a great success." Carter tapped the folders. "I'm not saying anything more. I was told to keep my mouth shut and I will."

"Don't make me get Natalie on you. Or better yet don't make me get your grandson on you. Because you know you'll lose."

Carter laughed. "Well even under that kind of duress I'll have to keep quiet." He stood and tucked the folders under his arm and walked to the door. "You'll find out soon enough. All I'll say for now is that the future looks very interesting—and promising for you."

Michael sat there after he left wondering what it was that he had alluded to and teased him about. He thought about speaking to the Secretary-General and what that could mean for the ULE. Without doubt, it could be used internationally. He thought of the fallout of what had happened in Europe during the Syrian refugee crisis. And how that situation was still stressing many governments. There is so much that could have been done differently. But it would take decision-makers that had a different framework and could look at things in a different context. Those kinds of leaders weren't in power back then. In the ULE was the means to provide that ability in leaders now and in the future. He thought about all the lives it would save and suffering it would prevent. He looked at his planner and appointment book. He picked up the phone and started his daily calls. He had a lot of work still to do.

* * *

A MONTH LATER
THE UNITED NATIONS
NEW YORK CITY

He stood there looking out on the General Assembly, seated in row after row, and a part of him still wondered at where he had come from and how he got to this place and time. He turned to Margot Akerstrom, who had just introduced him.

"Thank you, Madame Secretary. Ladies and gentlemen, it is an honor to talk to you today. The U.N. was started in 1957 as an international organization to help promote peace and stability in the world. Since its inception, the world has gone through many changes. There have been wars, the specter of nuclear annihilation, there has been genocide famines and now climate change. We are facing problems on a level that we have not faced before. But in some ways the more things change, the more things stay the same. Many of the same issues that the U.N. was formed to address are still prevalent. What I'm going to talk to you about today is the way to change some of our fundamental world problems."

He paused to sip from the glass of water on the low table next to the podium

"Ideas are what bring about change. The idea of democracy changed the world. Religious ideas have changed the world. But we still have serious problems worldwide not fixed by either of them. What I am going to talk to you about today is the idea—I'll emphasize that—the idea that will change, and improve, our world.

"Albert Einstein said that we can't solve problems by using the same kind of thinking we used when we created them. I believe that to be true. What I would like to invite you to do is to start thinking about some of these global problems in a different way.

"For most economic performance and industrialized nations, we judge success by a single measurement. The Gross Domestic Product (GDP) is the metric we use to determine if our country is in good, overall, shape. But is it really? I think that we need a measurement, a benchmark that covers far more than the country's economic performance. The interesting, and disturbing, truth is that rising wealth doesn't always equate to a good and happy society. There's a clear case — and this is certainly talked about a great deal over the last few years — that the rich get richer and the poor get poorer. So you can have a strong economy but most of the citizens are still badly off. That's not how it should be and we all know that. If a country, such as the United States, and its government and laws truly are for the people then that the government and the laws should provide some way of measuring how happy it citizens are.

"There's a new metric being used. One that I think is a very good tool to measure how successful a country actually is. There're twelve components to the index that covers the three basics of happy people which obviously leads to a happy society. Those are the basics of food, water, shelter, opportunity, freedom of choice, freedom from discrimination, and a chance for higher education. We all need the pillars of a basic education, healthcare and a safe, sustainable environment in which to live.

"Of the hundred and 133 countries evaluated in the index, the U.S. is ranked 16. Obviously being number 16 is better than any of the higher numbers. But I believe we can do much better and perhaps can even, not only in the United States but throughout the world, reach the point where we don't need to measure our success — our level of happiness — as much as we should appreciate and enjoy it.

"You have all read the reports on the ULE. In the last few years, we have diligently worked on educating the American public about it. The results: Our overall crime rate has gone down by 23%. Poverty has decreased by 21%. Our healthcare cost, once 17.6% of GDP is now 15.1%. By educating the people about the health benefits of the ULE, we have seen a 10.3% improvement in health in our country. Not too long ago the United States was ranked 37th, of developed countries, in infant mortality rate. Now we are ranked 3rd, and we expect to be ranked number one in the next two years. Some of this reduction is due to better science and reallocation of care. But much of it is due to different policies; policies that only became possible because of a change in the national viewpoint and a recognition that by helping the least of us, we help all of us.

"In a recent survey, where Americans were asked about their satisfaction with their lives in the country, they rated their satisfaction rate at 73%, whereas five or six years ago it was 54%. Using that as a barometer I would say the idea, and implementation of the ULE has improved the lives of citizens in the United States. America as a nation has embraced the ULE and has moved toward a country based more on cooperation than on competition. This has led to a significant improvement in the overall quality of the health and financial well-being of all Americans.

"We have a long way to go. We are not done. But we have been able, with the principles of the ULE, to make a fundamental change in the direction of our country and a radical improvement in the lives of the people.

"America is not alone in implementing the ULE. Other countries have taken notice and started to teach the ULE in their countries as well. We welcome these efforts. We stand ready to help in any way we can with any other country that would like to institute these changes and implement the ULE.

"What we have done in the United States of America can easily be implemented in still more countries. If you think about the history of mankind, civilization only started after individuals banded together and cooperated toward a mutually beneficial role. That goal at first was merely survival—the stability of basic needs such as enough food and shelter—and it grew more complex over thousands of years. We all know and can list many things wrong with the current state of our civilization. The shortcomings and challenges are too numerous to discuss her. Many think they are too complex to resolve. I think if we take away the tendency to overcomplicate things and to point at too many variables as being the root cause... that we can start with a very simple solution.

Cooperation. I suggest to you that if we do not cooperate that civilization will not solve the problems we face and that our world as we know it may cease to exist.

"I have written in the past about the ULE and the necessity to implement it if there is to be any chance of achieving universal peace. Clearly we cannot have that unless we strive to eliminate unnecessary resistance.

"The ULE can be the cornerstone of a new global society. But, and this is crucial, so please listen carefully to me. Whatever we choose as the underlying principle of our new society cannot be based on belief alone. We have tried that throughout history and it has not worked. One person may believe in one God the other person may believe in a different God and then there are people that do not believe in God at all.

"The ULE is not a matter of belief because it is proven with a mathematical theorem. A mathematical theory is not a matter of faith. Anyone who understands and is willing to follow the laws of logic would come to precisely the same conclusion. If we are to have a universal principle for how we maintain civilization, it has to be something we can all agree on. We all understand that systems—any system—functions most efficiently without unnecessary resistance. If we use the principles of the ULE and make every decision based on whether it increases or decreases resistance, then civilization will not only survive but thrive.

"Imagine a world where there is no war, where people feel safe and have enough to eat and all people live healthy, happy, productive lives. Given our world history, its wars and bloodshed, often fueled by intolerance, it may seem like this is an impossible dream. In the past it was. But we have evolved and learned and continue to do so. As children growing up, we learned that we cannot afford to think only of ourselves and not take the needs of others into account. As adults we need to return to that way of thinking. That must to be one of the goals of our continued maturation as global citizens.

"I said at the beginning of my speech, ideas change the world. The discovery of the ULE makes real global peace not only possible but inevitable. We now know what we need to do to create a better world. If we resolve to establish the ULE as the governing principle of our emerging global society, then civilization will flourish.

"I realize that this will not be easy. There will be people that only want to think of themselves. They will not embrace what I just told you; that by helping the least of us, we help all of us. They will challenge what we do and this idea and what it brings about—change—will be hard to accomplish. It should not deter us from this path. We owe it to ourselves and our children and indeed the survival of mankind to do this. There is no other choice. Thank you."

EPILOGUE

We are crying for a vision. That all living things can share. And those who care are with us everywhere.
—Kate Wolf, Brother Warrior

TWO YEARS LATER

Washington DC | AP NewsWire

The U.S. Senate overwhelmingly confirmed U.S. President Allan Benton's choice of Senator Michael Wharton (I) Colorado, currently serving his second term, to be Secretary of State, with Republicans and Democrats praising him as the ideal successor to James Winston Ericcson. Wharton, by far, becomes the youngest Secretary of State in the history of the United States of America.

The vote Tuesday was 94-3. One senator — Wharton — voted present and accepted congratulations from colleagues on the Senate floor. The roll call came just hours after the Senate Foreign Relations Committee unanimously approved the man who has led the panel for the past year and was instrumental in creating and implementing a nationwide program predicated on individual improvement as the basis for improving every facet of life in our nation.

No date has been set for Wharton's swearing-in though a welcoming ceremony is planned at the State Department on Monday.

* * *

"A tiny thing is Man, on the scale of the Universe, but in some people their soul is the Universe."
—Dennis Lowery

We are all small in the grand scheme of things, but some have within us the power to make our reality

The Unlocked Soul

much larger... much more complete and to our liking. We see not just who we are, but who we can become. We appreciate what we have, yet still reach toward a goal or objective. Stretching ourselves.

Those of us who were not born perfect know that each day of our life is an opportunity to learn more, do more and be more. Even if it's only a small step, a bit of progress or when your personal circle of enlightenment expands slightly to push back the shadows and darkness of the path ahead and that borders the sides of the road we travel in life.

Invictus

(William Ernest Henley, 1849–1903)

Out of the night that covers me,
Black as the pit from pole to pole,
I thank whatever gods may be
For my unconquerable soul.

In the fell clutch of circumstance
I have not winced nor cried aloud.
Under the bludgeonings of chance
My head is bloody but unbowed.

Beyond this place of wrath and tears
Looms but the Horror of the shade,
And yet the menace of the years
Finds and shall find me unafraid.

Jonathan Berman

It matters not how strait the gate,
How charged with punishments the scroll,
I am the master of my fate:
I am the captain of my soul.

ABOUT THE AUTHORS

Jonathan Berman

Jonathan holds a BS in Mathematics and a MS in Statistics. When finishing his undergraduate degree in mathematics he discovered a mathematical theorem that proves the universal law discussed in this book. The Universal Law of Efficiency has profound implications for human health and longevity, human evolution, and universal peace.

Jonathan became aware of how tension affects the body at the young age of 20. Over the course of the next year, through various methods including stretching and meditation, he got to a point of almost no tension in his body. Jonathan's life purpose has been a journey of reducing tension in his own body and helping other people reduce the tension in their bodies and other systems.

Jonathan has studied yoga, ballet, and other physical and meditative practices since 1978. Jonathan has a private healing practice and teaches classes on the healing benefits of the Universal Law of Efficiency.

Jonathan and his wife, Erin, continue to work on getting this information out to the world because it has tremendous implications for humanity.

Erin Whitney

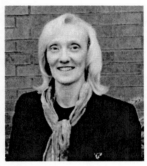 Erin holds a BS in Business Management and an MA in Clinical Psychology. After 10 years in the business field in New York and Chicago, since 1998 she has worked in clinical, non-profit, hospital, home, and school settings as a Licensed Professional Counselor.

In addition to counseling, Ms. Whitney currently works as a Life Coach, True Purpose® Coach, Transitions Coach, Career Coach and Spiritual Coach.

Ms. Whitney has been a presenter and Advanced Trainer for educators, parents and clinicians in The Nurtured Heart Approach® since 2003, and has worked with Jonathan Berman for over 9 years to help articulate the Universal Law of Efficiency. Jon and Erin have enjoyed a happy and fulfilling marriage since 2010.

Ms. Whitney has had an interest in working to help people live more peacefully for as long as she can remember. Her own personal growth work since 1998 and her ongoing spiritual education, as well as her formal education and experience, have influenced her to focus on ways to help people cooperatively live their most fulfilled, peaceful and enlightened lives. Living the Universal Law of Efficiency and helping others to understand it are major ways she helps create a peaceful, healthy and fulfilling existence for everyone.

ABOUT THE UNIVERSAL LAW OF EFFICIENCY

Some people have said that profound truths are very simple.

This paper discusses a Universal Truth that has been proven by a mathematical theorem. The Universal Law of Efficiency™ (ULE) states that all systems function most efficiently without unnecessary resistance. Since human beings are systems, human beings function most efficiently without unnecessary resistance. Most if not all systems, contain necessary, unnecessary, and inherent resistance.

The Theorem

One of the values of mathematics is that it is a synthetic system that can prove universal truths given certain assumptions. The Efficiency Theorem (ET) assumes that there is such a thing as systems and that systems function more or less efficiently based on a frame of reference. Because mathematics is based on logic rather than empirical evidence, scientific studies are not needed to prove that a theorem is true. Once proven, a theorem will always be true, regardless of changes in society or worldviews.

The Unlocked Soul

Because mathematical theorems prove universal truths, ideas based on theorems must be taken seriously. The ET proves the ULE, which applies to all systems.

The ET states that all systems function most efficiently without unnecessary resistance.

Definitions:

System – a set of interrelated parts forming a complex whole.

Unnecessary Resistance – That which impedes the accomplishment of a goal or objective.

Necessary Resistance -That which is required to accomplish a goal or objective.

Inherent Resistance – Resistance in a system that cannot be classified as either necessary or unnecessary.

The Proof

The ET is proven using a proof by contradiction. A proof by contradiction assumes the opposite of what one wants to prove and demonstrates that that assumption leads to a contradiction.

The proof of the ET is as follows. Assume that there exists some system that functions most efficiently with unnecessary resistance. But then it wouldn't be unnecessary. Therefore, all systems function most efficiently without unnecessary resistance.

The proof of the ET relies on the fact that there are only two possible cases where systems can function most efficiently, and one and only one of those cases can be true. The first case is that all systems function most efficiently without unnecessary resistance. The second case is that there exists at least one system that functions most efficiently with unnecessary resistance.

The ET could be disproven by demonstrating that there exists at least one system that functions most efficiently with unnecessary resistance. Since the goal is to prove that all systems function most efficiently without unnecessary resistance, the proof starts by assuming that there exists at least one system that functions most efficiently with unnecessary resistance. Since it is clearly a contradiction to have a system that functions most efficiently with unnecessary resistance, it must be true that all systems function most efficiently without unnecessary resistance.

The ET proves that the ULE is true for all systems

A categorical syllogism can be used to demonstrate that the ULE applies to human beings. A categorical syllogism is an "argument consisting of exactly three categorical propositions (two premises and a conclusion) in which there appears a total of exactly three categorical terms, each of which is used exactly twice."(Kemerling, 2006) More specifically, an AAA-1 syllogism is used which has the following form:

- All F are R.
- All A are F.
- Therefore, all A are R.
- Although all syllogisms of this form are valid, both premises must be correct for the conclusion to be correct. The following syllogism is valid, but the conclusion is incorrect.
- All fruits are red.
- All apples are fruits.
- Therefore, all apples are red.
- It is not true that all fruits are red. This leads to the erroneous conclusion that all apples are red.
- The syllogism that relates the ULE to human beings is as follows:
- All systems function most efficiently without unnecessary resistance.
- All human beings are systems.
- Therefore, all human beings function most efficiently without unnecessary resistance.

The first premise is the ULE. Since it was proven, it must be correct.

The second premise is correct by definition. The definition of a system is "a set of connected things or parts forming a complex whole. Physiology – the human or animal body as a whole."(Oxford University Press Inc., 2006)

Since the first two premises of the syllogism are true, it follows that the conclusion must be true; that all human beings function most efficiently without unnecessary resistance.

An example should help to make this clear. Suppose someone is riding a bicycle uphill and wants to get up the hill as easily as possible. Putting the brakes on would create unnecessary resistance. If someone is riding a bicycle toward a precipice and doesn't want to die, putting the brakes on would be necessary resistance.

These examples illustrate that there can be both necessary and unnecessary resistance in the same system at different times. What is necessary or unnecessary resistance in a system depends on the frame of reference from which the system is viewed. This is an important point, particularly when considering how the ULE relates to human health.

By frame of reference, I mean how you look at a particular situation. As human beings, we always have a choice as to how we look at things. Time is an important factor in how we perceive a particular situation. There are times when a short term perspective is very important, such as when a person is about to be hit by a bus, and times when a longer term perspective is more important. Different time frames can be parameters in the "decision matrix" used to determine whether something is necessary or unnecessary resistance in a human system.

The total resistance in a system can be expressed in the formula: $R_t = R_u + R_n + R_i$

Where R_t is the total resistance, R_u is unnecessary resistance, R_n is necessary resistance, and R_i is inherent resistance. In the example of riding a bicycle uphill, R_u is putting the brakes on, R_n is the resistance of the bicycle chain on the gears, and R_i is the force of gravity. It is difficult to categorize gravity as either necessary or unnecessary, but it affects the system.

It is possible that unnecessary resistance is a large percentage of the total resistance in human beings. If true, eliminating the unnecessary resistance from human beings would go a long way toward helping people function more efficiently.

Unnecessary resistance in a human being is unnecessary holding which manifests as unnecessary tension. Clenching your fist takes a lot of effort, and unless you are doing so for particular reason, it is unnecessary tension and resistance.

Most people are unaware of how much tension they have in their bodies, nor how much better life would be without it. Better physical and emotional health, greater clarity of thought, and more compassion for ourselves and others are some of the benefits of getting the tension out of our bodies. Holding tension takes energy that could be better used for other things such as overcoming disease.

Getting all of the unnecessary tension out of the body means that all the vertebrae are optimally aligned and there is no unnecessary compression or distortion in the body. It also means letting go of all held emotions, such as fear or sadness, which usually cause systemic tension. A person may be flexible enough to do the Chinese splits, but not have all of the unnecessary tension out of their body.

Everything we do in life either increases or decreases tension. This is true because everything in life changes, including the amount of tension we hold in our bodies. This self-evident truth is an important concept in how the ULE relates to human beings.

The Implications

The ULE has many implications for human beings and other systems. These implications include biomechanical, medical, and psychological applications and how we relate to one another in relationships, families, communities, and societies. It also has implications for the next step in human evolution and our view of the nature of reality.

There are innumerable instances where getting all of the unnecessary tension out of the body can be helpful. This paper will focus on physical and psychological health benefits, the implications for human evolution, and the benefits to society.

The Health Benefits

It is clear that all bodily functions work better if the body is working most efficiently. In particular, a person would be healthier if the body were working more efficiently rather than less efficiently. This suggests a new definition of disease could be that a body is not functioning efficiently enough to fight off germs, viruses, or other foreign bodies. More specifically, disease is a function of the body's inability to maintain homeostasis. "Homeostasis is the body's maintenance of a stable internal environment; it is so important that most of our metabolic energy is spent on it." (David Shier, 2004)

The Physics

In the discussion that follows, the term "energy" will be used solely in the sense that physicists use the term. The term "chi" is often used in traditional Chinese medicine and it connotes a particular type of "life force", or animating principle that differentiates us from inanimate objects such as stones or metal.

Let's try a thought experiment. Assume that two engines are the same in every detail except that the first engines bearings, rings, and cylinders are perfectly adjusted and machined for optimum performance while the second engines bearing are too tight and the pistons and rings are slightly large for the cylinders. The laws of physics guarantee that, all else being equal, the first engine will last longer and perform better than the second engine. This is because the first engine has less resistance and, therefore, works more efficiently. The ULE guarantees that all systems, be they engines or human beings, function most efficiently without unnecessary resistance.

The same laws of physics that apply to engines apply to human beings. The more resistance there is in a human body, the less efficiently that body will work. Unnecessary resistance in a human being is caused by unnecessary tension.

"It takes a good portion of the body's metabolic energy to maintain homeostasis." (David Shier, 2004) Since the energy it takes to hold tension in the body is no longer available to help maintain homeostasis, the body will not be as efficient in fighting off a disease or repairing a wound. Theoretically, if the body had instantaneous access to unlimited amounts of energy, it could fight off any disease, and the average human lifespan would be greatly increased.

A person in a Sympathetic Nervous System response of "Fight or Flight or Freeze", (FFF) uses a lot of energy to deal with an immediate threat. This causes a net energy loss which must be repaid. Doctors recommend that sick people get plenty of rest. This allows the body to use its energy mainly to fight off disease. If a person is in FFF while sick, their ability to heal will be impaired. Since held emotions often involve FFF, these held emotions impair a person's ability to heal. Other held or current emotions such as anger and sadness have the same effect.

There can be little doubt that there is a mind-body connection. If a person a sees someone pointing a gun at them, there will be a noticeable change in the body chemistry. If a person sees a *shadow* that they think is someone pointing a gun at them, they will experience the same effect.

Our worldviews affect our bodies. The "placebo effect" bears this out. It has been shown that if a person believes that they are taking a drug that will help them, they will sometimes heal regardless of whether they are taking a drug or not. The interesting question is why this works and what it says about the nature of reality. If belief can cause the body to heal, can a negative belief or thought pattern cause disease?

Since there is a mind-body connection, it follows that a person's worldview can affect their health. Deeply held systemic tension is usually caused by held emotions, beliefs, or experiences.

When a person gets hit physically or emotionally, muscles clench to avoid feeling pain. Adults usually have the ability to release situational tension with no lasting effects. Young children, however, are not so fortunate.

Young children absorb the conscious and unconscious emotions and programming of their parents and environment. This programming can take the form of one or both parents consciously or subconsciously demanding that the child shut down part of their body or spirit because of the parents' unresolved issues. Young children cannot separate their parents' issues from reality. For the young child, their parents' worldview is reality, and taking on that programming is a matter of survival; it is necessary tension. It can also take the form of environmental stressors such as sexual abuse. As a grown up, the holding on once needed to survive becomes unnecessary tension.

People are often unaware of the specific emotions or experiences they hold in their bodies. Held experiences usually have an FFF component and are an on-going energy drain. Long-term contraction of muscles inhibits the circulation of blood, oxygen, and chi, which eventually leads to disease or musculoskeletal problems.

The Progression of a Disease

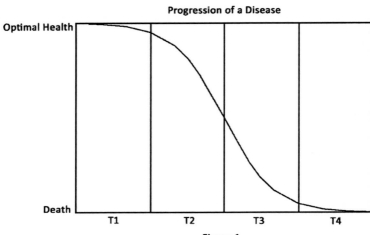

Figure 1

Diseases such as cancer do not manifest instantaneously. The progression from optimal health to death can typically be graphed as a sigmoidal curve. Figure 1 above shows an idealized graph of the progression of a disease, assuming no intervention. In real life, the graph of a disease may not be symmetrical and the distribution of T_1 through T_4 may be unequal. T_1 represents the onset of a disease. During nascency, maintaining homeostasis does not require substantial extra energy. During T_2, the rate of growth of malignant cells increases exponentially. At this stage, the body needs substantially more energy to successfully fight off a disease. During T_3, the rate of growth of malignant cells slows and the defenses of the affected part of the body are almost fully overwhelmed. By T_4, the bodily functions start to shut down and death occurs.

Since a disease can only progress beyond nascency if the body is incapable of maintaining homeostasis, it makes sense to have as much energy available as possible to fight off a disease at the onset. This suggests that people should strive to release tension from their bodies to maintain homeostasis and stay healthy.

Chi and Health

The unnecessary tension in the body not only affects blood and oxygen circulation but also affects how chi flows in the body. Traditional Chinese medicine holds that disease is usually caused by blocked chi in the body. Getting the unnecessary tension out of the body allows the body to relaxed, and the chi to flow more freely. If the chi flows more freely, healing occurs.

Unlike car engines, human beings have the ability to heal. Eliminating the cause of a disease can eliminate the effect. Discovering and releasing the causes of tension allows the chi to flow and the body to heal.

Techniques for Releasing Tension

As stated above, everything we do in life either increases or decreases tension. Releasing tension from the body involves doing more things that release tension and fewer things that increase tension. There are many methods of releasing tension including yoga, tai chi, meditation, and others.

Releasing deep systemic tension usually requires getting in touch with long-held emotions. This allows the body to release which frees up the energy to maintain homeostasis and allows the chi to flow.

Case Study

Patricia (not her real name) is a 70-year-old woman who had Lyme Disease for two years. She was in a lot of pain and could not walk. After six one-hour phone sessions using techniques to release unnecessary tension and resistance, Patricia could walk again and was 60% pain-free. Each session involved looking at her old held issues or "pictures." One picture was of her as a young girl where she was kneeling on the ground with both of her parents pushing down on a board on top of her. The picture was a representation of a psychological dynamic that existed between Patricia and her parents. By getting in touch with the emotions the picture represented, we were able to release the tension which allowed her chi to flow more freely.

While the ULE doesn't require empirical evidence because it was proven by the ET, more research is needed to substantiate the effectiveness of the above methods.

Treating cancer using these techniques would be significantly less damaging than radiation therapy. Assuming that both modalities had the same probability of success, many people might choose the former.

There are many diseases or conditions, where getting the excess tension out of the body would be helpful purely from a biomechanical perspective. Musculoskeletal conditions such as scoliosis or lordosis could be helped by releasing unnecessary tension.

High blood pressure is a big problem in this country. Blood vessels are semi-permeable capillaries. If the muscles around vessels are tight, the blood vessel is compressed, which reduces the cross-sectional area. This means that the heart has to work harder to get the same amount of blood to flow in a compressed space. Equations in physics describe the mathematical relationship of how compressing a volume of fluid into a smaller volume increases the pressure in that fluid.

High blood pressure can be caused by plaque buildup inside of blood vessels. This buildup reduces the cross-sectional area of the blood vessel, which raises the blood pressure. Reducing tension in the body may not directly affect the buildup of plaque, but it will increase the cross-sectional area of blood vessels, which will lower the blood pressure.

Reducing the overall tension in our bodies could go a long way toward reducing the prevalence of high blood pressure in our society.

The ULE and Psychology

The ULE and the methods described above could be used to treat psychological disorders as well as physical diseases. It has been suggested that the ULE is the unifying principle that links all psychological treatment modalities.

The existence of a mind-body connection and the implications of the ULE suggest that psychological and physical health is inextricably linked. Improving mental health by releasing held emotions or traumatic experiences reduces tension in the body. This increases the energy available for maintaining homeostasis and allows blood, oxygen, and chi to flow more freely. This improves physical health. Based on ULE, doctors may become more concerned with a patient's emotional health.

There are times when treating a disease or injury may initially require the techniques of Western medicine. Incorporating methods of releasing held emotions, however, could shorten the recovery period and reduce the need for extensive medication. The ULE should be part of any psychological/physical treatment plan.

The ET and Health Costs in Society

According to the National Health Expenditure Accounts which are the official estimates of total health care spending in the United States, in 2009 total health expenditures reached $2.5 trillion, or 17.6 percent of the nation's GDP. (U.S. Department of Health and Human Services, 2011)

If the awareness and implementation of the ET improved the overall health in this country by 1%, it would save the country approximately 25 billion dollars per year. If the government invested one billion dollars in educating the public and training practitioners, there would be a considerable return on investment. Even if there were only a billion-dollar savings in the first year, there would likely be an exponential increase in savings in subsequent years.

This approach to treating disease would be relatively inexpensive. It does not require expensive drugs or technology. Also, it would take much less time and money to train health care providers to use these techniques than it does to train medical doctors. Because this method is low tech, it could be used in areas with substandard medical facilities such as 3rd world countries.

The ULE and Human Evolution

Getting all of the unnecessary tension out of the body is a major step in human evolution both physically and emotionally. Evolution is a change in a species which allows the species to function more efficiently in an environment. Getting the unnecessary tension out of our bodies would allow human beings to function more efficiently in every way that makes us human.

Getting the unnecessary tension out of the body would enhance human performance, particularly in sports. Since muscles move bones, asymmetrical tension causes spinal misalignment. To understand the problem, try to run while holding your hips to one side. The body functions most efficiently if bones are optimally aligned, which can only happen if there is no unnecessary tension. Tension reduces the energy available for activities such as running a race.

Most people would agree that a person would think more clearly with less tension rather than more tension in their head. I can easily think five moves ahead in chess if there is no unnecessary tension in my head. A small increase in the intellectual ability of people in the world would have a profound effect on sciences, the arts, technology and the environment.

Some people have suggested that technology has surpassed our emotional development. The specter of nuclear war makes this a frightening prospect. Releasing held emotions would allow us to evolve emotionally which makes global perspectives more attainable. The more we base our actions on universal principles rather than immediate emotional needs, the better off we will be. Widespread implementation of the ULE would increase our chances of having a future.

The ULE and Society

The ULE applies to all systems. Since societies are systems, societies function most efficiently without unnecessary resistance. The goal of all societies, religions, and spiritual practices is to make things work more efficiently from some frame of reference.

The ULE provides a non-dogmatic paradigm for human interaction. Once one understands that everything we do in life either increases or decreases tension, enlightened self-interest suggests that doing things that increase tension – such as lying, raping or killing – is contra-productive. Yelling or getting angry takes a lot of energy. Raping somebody could create tremendous guilt in the rapist, which will eventually lead to physical and/or psychological illness. As people become more aware of this dynamic, they will be more conscious of their actions. It is nice to know that doing something that is good for us, such as releasing unnecessary tension, ultimately helps the world. Since the ET is a theorem, it provides a framework for people to judge their actions that are not based on belief or subject to change.

Because the ULE is a universal law, it is something that everyone can agree on. Regardless of whether one is an atheist, Buddhist, Christian, Jew or Muslin, one cannot dispute the ULE. Focusing on our commonalities rather than perceived differences will bring the human race closer together. We are less likely go to war with people that are the same as us rather than different.

We are rapidly developing a world culture that may transcend cultural, ethnic, and religious differences. This will require universal principles that we can all agree upon and live by. The ULE is just such a principle.

Teaching the concepts of the ULE in schools would be invaluable. If children are taught that everything we do in life either increases or decreases tension and that yelling or hitting other children will negatively affect them, they will find other methods of getting their needs met. Children are generally egocentric and will do what they perceive to be in their own best interests. If children grow up with a thorough understanding of the ULE, it will have a tremendously beneficial effect on society.

As Michael Guillen points out in his book "*Five Mathematical Equations that Changed the World*", once we understood the mathematics of flight, "It took us only fifty years to go from soaring above Kitty Hawk to soaring into space." (Guillen, 1995) Once we understand the underlying principle of the ULE, we will soar into a better world.

Bibliography

- David Shier, J. B. (2004). *Hole's Anatomy and Physiology*. New York: McGraw-Hill.

- Guillen, M. (1995). *Five Equations that Changed the World: The Power and Poetry of Mathematics.* New York: Hyperion.
- Kemerling, G. (2006, October 18). *Philosophy Pages.* Retrieved January 1, 2011, from http://www.philosophypages.com/lg/e08a.htm
- Oxford University Press Inc. (2006). *Concise Oxford American Dictionary.* New York: Oxford University Press Inc.
- U.S. Department of Health and Human Services. (2011, January 20). *National Health Expenditures 2009 Highlights.* Retrieved February 1, 2011, from Historical National Health Expenditure Data: https://www.cms.gov/NationalHealthExpendData/downloads/highlight.pdf

The Role of Mathematics in Human Knowledge

In the past, we relied on observation to gain knowledge about the world. For example, people saw that if they left meat out and did not cook it, eventually maggots would appear. This led to a view of reality that was the best they could come up with at the time, given the tools they had to work with.

Eventually, these natural observations, albeit often wrong, were codified into written texts and became what we call religion. As we gained better tools such as telescopes and microscopes, we gained a better understanding of how the world really works. Microscopes lead to the discovery of germs and microbial contaminants and how they affect health.

Mathematics provides a way of proving things that even science is not capable of. Even the most fervid religious devotee relies on the laws of physics when taking a plane ride. Similarly, they also believe and expect that law of gravity will apply to them if they jump off the edge of a cliff. Mathematics relies on logic rather than empirical evidence to prove something. While some people still question whether global warming is real, no one can question the Pythagorean Theorem. Different branches of mathematics are based on different assumptions. Euclidean geometry is based on the assumption that parallel lines do not meet in infinity and that planes are "flat". Once one assumes these axioms, one can prove things based on those assumptions. Since mathematics is a synthetic system, it can prove things within certain tautological limits. But it is the only system that can truly prove universal concepts. For example, there are infinitely many right triangles. The Pythagorean Theorem states that for ALL right triangles in Euclidean space, $a^2 + b^2 = c^2$. The techniques of science cannot prove this. It would be impossible to measure with infinite accuracy all of the infinitely many right triangles in the Universe. Only mathematics can prove that $a^2 + b^2 = c^2$.

Scientific Method is a very powerful technique, but it relies on empirical evidence. Galileo observed the motion of the sun and moon and deduced that the world was not flat and that the world was not the center of the universe.

It is passed time that we require a higher level of proof regarding how we view the world.

Yoga, Mathematics, and Human Evolution

Most people are unaware of how much tension they have in their bodies, nor how much better life would be without it. Better physical and emotional health, greater clarity of thought, and more compassion for ourselves and others are some of the benefits of getting the tension out of our bodies.

When I was twenty, I was so tight I felt I would die from the tension in three or four days. My body felt cold and numb and everything inside was black. I avoided experiencing emotions such as anger, fear, sadness, and guilt, by not being in my body.

If you have only four days left to live, you have some stark choices to make. You do what it takes to stay alive or you decide to die. I decided to do what it took to stay alive. Over the next year and a half, I did a lot of meditating and stretching to get in touch withheld emotions and gets my energy or chi flowing. I got to where there was only a tiny bit of tension in my center, the *uddiyana bandha*. That tension was the only separation between Self and Not-Self. I felt that I would turn into an energy field and disappear if I let go of that tension. Most people are neither as tense as I was when I was twenty nor as free from tension as I was in the following year, but most people can benefit much more than they know from releasing tension from the body.

Several years ago, while finishing my Bachelors in Mathematics, I discovered a theorem that proves the benefits of releasing tension from the body. The Efficiency Theorem states that "All systems function most efficiently without unnecessary resistance in the system." (If you doubt this, ask yourself if any system functions most efficiently *with* unnecessary resistance.)

Most systems need some resistance to function. This is necessary resistance. If you are riding a bicycle toward a precipice, putting the brakes on is necessary resistance. If you are riding uphill, putting the brakes on is unnecessary resistance. The goal of the system defines what is necessary or unnecessary.

Since human beings are systems, human beings function most efficiently without unnecessary resistance. What is unnecessary resistance in a human being? Unnecessary tension.

When I talk about unnecessary tension, I mean both tension that we can feel that makes it uncomfortable to sit in full lotus, and deeper tension that we cannot feel that distorts the spine and keeps the vertebrae from "floating" on one another. I could do the Chinese splits long before I got all the tension out of my hips. People that have all of the tension out of their bodies literally glow, so much that they light up a dark room at night. They also have totally open hearts.

Clenching your fist for any length of time makes you realize that holding tension takes effort. As the Efficiency Theorem proves, tension makes the body perform less efficiently. Would you think more clearly with more or less tension in your head?

The heart has less room to expand if there is tension in the chest and so has to beat faster to pump the same amount of blood. Tension in the body constricts blood vessels which make the heart work harder still. Think of trying to move water through a kinked hose.

Long-term contraction of muscles inhibits the circulation of both blood and energy, which eventually leads to disease and musculoskeletal problems. Deeply held systemic tension is usually caused by held emotions, beliefs, or experiences. When a person gets hit physically or emotionally, muscles clench to avoid feeling pain. Adults usually have the ability to release situational tension with no lasting effects. Young children, however, are not so fortunate.

Young children absorb the conscious and unconscious emotions and programming of their parents and environment. This programming can take the form of one or both parents consciously or subconsciously demanding that the child shut down part of their body or spirit because of the parents' unresolved issues. Young children cannot separate their parents' issues from reality. For the young child, their parents' worldview *is* reality, and taking on that programming is a matter of survival; it is necessary tension. As a grown up, the tension once needed for survival becomes unnecessary tension.

People continue to hold on to old programming and emotions through fear or lack of knowledge. Students often tell me that they are always tight in some part of their bodies. When I ask them why, they often do not have an answer. Knowledge makes holding onto emotions a choice. Getting in touch withheld emotions is, for me, the hardest part of yoga. Releasing emotions takes time, courage and compassion, but the benefits are definitely worth the effort.

Reducing tension in the body greatly enhances human performance, particularly in sports. Since muscles move bones, asymmetrical tension causes spinal misalignment. To understand the problem, try to run while holding your hips to one side. The body functions most efficiently if bones are optimally aligned, which can only happen if there is no unnecessary tension. Also, tension reduces the energy available for other activities such as running a race.

I use techniques of getting in touch withheld emotions to heal myself and others. Traditional Chinese medicine teaches that illness is caused by blocked chi. Getting in touch with held emotions allows muscles to release and chi to flow more freely. As the chi flows more freely, the body becomes healthier. Eliminating the cause eliminates the effect.

I recently worked with a woman who had Lyme Disease and could barely walk. After six sessions, to help her release tension and held emotions, she could walk again, had much more energy, and 70% less pain. Helping her experience deeply held negative "pictures" or beliefs that she was unaware of allowed her energy to flow and fostered better health. All bodily processes – including staying healthy – work best if the body is working most efficiently.

Getting all of the unnecessary tension out of the body is a major step in human evolution. Evolution is a change in a species which allows the species to function more efficiently in an environment. Getting the unnecessary tension out of our bodies allows human beings to function more efficiently in every way that makes us human.

The Efficiency Theorem also suggests a non-dogmatic paradigm for human interaction. Once one understands that everything we do in life either increases or decreases tension, enlightened self-interest suggests that doing things that increase tension – such as lying, raping or killing – is contra-productive. For example, raping somebody could create tremendous guilt in the rapist, which will eventually lead to physical and/or psychological illness. As people become more aware of this dynamic, they will be more conscious of their actions. The Efficiency Theorem provides a framework for people to judge their actions that are not based on belief or subject to change.

Jonathan Berman

As Michael Guillen points out in his book *"The Five Mathematical Equations that Changed the World"*, once we understood how airplanes really flew, "It took us only fifty years to go from soaring above Kitty Hawk to soaring into space" (p. 117). Once we understand how tension affects us, we will soar into a better world.

At the highest level, releasing unnecessary tension is releasing foundational beliefs such as the belief in time and space. Fear of letting go of these beliefs has kept me from releasing that final point of tension; the last separation between Self and Not-Self. As we evolve toward less tension, we evolve toward greater Enlightenment.

CPSIA information can be obtained
at www.ICGtesting.com
Printed in the USA
FSOW02n0757060416
18837FS